The Immunology of Human Pregnancy

Contemporary Biomedicine

The Immunology
of Human Pregnancy

Henry N. Claman

University of Colorado Health Sciences Center,

Denver, Colorado

Humana Press • **Totowa, New Jersey**

Dedication

Dedicated to the memories of Leoni Neumann Claman, MD and Irving Claman, MD, practitioners of "the old school." They would have been intrigued by the parts of this book they understood, and would have been proud of the other parts because they were written by their son.

© 1993 The Humana Press Inc.
999 Riverview Dr., Suite 208
Totowa, New Jersey 07512

Printed in the United States of America. 10 9 8 7 6 5 4 3 2 1

Library of Congress Cataloging in Publication Data
Claman, Henry N., 1930–
      The immunology of human pregnancy / Henry N. Claman.
          p. cm. (Contemporary biomedicine)
      Includes index.
      ISBN 0-89603-251-5
      1. Pregnancy—Immunological aspects. I. Title.
      [DNLM: 1. Maternal–Fetal Exchange—immunology. 2. Pregnancy—
—immunology.   WQ 200 C586i]
RG557.C5 1993
612.6'3—dc20
DNLM/DLC
for Library of Congress   92-49012
                                                CIP

Preface

This book grew out of my interest in what is often called "the immunological paradox of pregnancy." How is it possible that the fetus—half of whose genetic apparatus comes from the father and is foreign to the mother—can survive to term? This is a question that intrigues all immunologists. For me, it has been of interest ever since I heard a lecture on the subject in medical school, long before I thought of becoming a "professional immunologist." Indeed, the question of the immunological aspect of fetal survival (or demise) should be of interest to any biologist or physician. The question becomes broader if one considers the immunologic relations between mother and fetus, because they represent a unique symbiotic union. What immunologic problems in the mother may affect the offspring, and is it possible that fetal immunology will affect the mother? Finally, there is the question of whether immunology is important in recurrent spontaneous abortion.

Every author owes the reader a general oversight of the book in hand, indicating the terrain to be covered, and, by inference, the territory that will not be explored.

1. This is primarily a book for clinicians. I will only mention animal experiments and data in passing, and as they may illuminate a clinical problem or observation.
2. The interest here is the immunology of materno–fetal relations, once a pregnancy has begun. Therefore, I will not cover immunological aspects of sterility, nor touch on the immunological approaches to controlling fertility, i.e., "contraceptive vaccines."
3. This is a book mainly concerned with pathogenesis. Thus it will not dwell on strictly clinical aspects of pregnancy itself, nor with the regular features of par-

ticular autoimmune syndromes. These topics are well covered in available textbooks.

4. AIDS presents a particular challenge to the student of pregnancy. Today, however, that field is generally understood in terms of infectious disease, rather than immunology itself. As such, I will not cover it. Besides, the field of AIDS research is moving so rapidly that any material on the subject that was prepared for this book would be hopelessly outdated by the time of publication.

5. Immunodeficiencies and infectious diseases affecting the mother and fetus are again best approached from the infectious disease standpoint. I will consider this topic mainly in terms of the general immunocompetence of the pregnant woman.

It is obvious that the book could have been much larger. In the interest of economy of time, and because of my wish to make this an integrated book with a single (if tolerant) viewpoint, I have chosen to be somewhat selective in my approach.

I have also been selective in reviewing and citing the available literature. Not every paper on every topic, no matter how relevant, is mentioned. Some publications are clearly redundant, some have been superseded, and others may best be left undisturbed.

As to classification, this book falls between traditional rubrics. It is not a textbook on immunology, and so a sophisticated immunologist will find Chapter 1—my overview of current immunology—understated. It is not a textbook on obstetrics or perinatal medicine, and so sophisticated obstetricians and pediatricians prefer more from Chapter 2. Perhaps it might be best to consider this volume as a hybrid, like the fetomaternal unit itself, participating equally in the life of pregnancy and the world of immunology.

I am grateful to many people for the help they have provided. Thanks go to my chairmen, Robert Schrier and Lewis Pizer, for letting me take a brief sabbatical and to Stephen Dreskin for so capably handling my duties during that time. I am deeply thankful to the Rockefeller Foundation for selecting me as a Resident Scholar so that I could write the first draft of this book during a stay at the Rockefeller Study and Conference Center, Bellagio, Italy. I thank Gungor Eroglu, who stimulated my interest in the problem of recurrent spontaneous abortion. I had helpful discussions with Gerald Chaouat, J.-F. Bach, and Guy Voisin, all in Paris. This book would not have been possible without encouragement and constructive criticism from my wife, Janet Stewart, although at times she may have heard more on the subject than she thought necessary. Finally, I am grateful to Kathryn Utschinski for creative manuscript preparation, and for her patience when I asked her to make room for "just one more reference."

Prologue

The Question

I am relatively certain that the main reason scientists study the immunology of pregnancy is because they are intrigued by *the immunological paradox of pregnancy.* They want to know the answer to the following question. *What mechanisms have developed that allow a genetically and immunologically foreign fetus to survive to term?* There are indeed other questions involving pregnancy and immunology that are not trivial. They include those about immunological aspects of infertility and sterility, infectious diseases in pregnancy, immunodeficiency syndromes in the fetus and newborn, AIDS in pregnancy, the development of vaccines for population control, and so forth. However, this book will concentrate on the paradox, and explore the immunological aspects of recurrent spontaneous abortion as a topic possibly related to the paradox.

It is not surprising that interest in the paradox grew apace during the great explosion of knowledge in immunology that occurred in the 1940–1960 period. During this time, the nature of cellular and humoral immune mechanisms was explored to a degree that was hitherto impossible. Of relevance to the paradox were the great strides taken in the field of tissue transplantation, a field led by the late Sir Peter Medawar.

Therefore, it is also no surprise that the landmark intellectual paper concerning the paradox came from Medawar himself. This paper carries the rather formidable title, *"Some Immunological and Endocrinological Problems Raised by the Evolution of Viviparity in Vertebrates."* Although it was published in a somewhat hard-to-find symposium series,[1] it has been very influential. One can read it for pleasure and for instruction today, not only for its insights but for the style of Medawar's prose—at the same time both magisterial and vivid.

Medawar gives three possible reasons "why the foetus does not habitually provoke an immunological reaction from its mother":

1. The anatomical separation of fetus from mother;
2. The antigenic immaturity of the fetus; and
3. The immunological indolence or inertness of the mother.

In discussing these reasons, Medawar marshaled evidence from various quarters, including both animal and human biology. He was greatly intrigued by the effects of hormones on allograft behavior and—rather surprising from the viewpoint of the 1990s—attributed the major role in fetal protection to "the enhanced secretion of cortisone-like steroids in pregnancy." That Medawar chose adrenocorticosteroids as major players in fetal protection comes from his own experimental work in rabbits that showed that corticosteroids have very potent antigraft activities in that species. That explanation does not seem to be true in humans, but this fact should not detract from Medawar's pioneering and insightful paper.

It appears that the intellectual mantle of Medawar, in terms of pregnancy immunology, then descended on the shoulders of Rupert E. Billingham. "Bill," as he is known to his colleagues, performed the most exacting and intriguing experiments in transplantation and reproductive immunology not only by himself, but with many able colleagues such as Willys K. Silvers and Alan E. Beer. These investigators were especially interested in "immunologically privileged sites." Billingham also had a gift for prose, and it is a pleasure to read his superb reviews even today.[2-4]

As the field of pregnancy immunology matured, it was clear that contributions would continue to come from both the animal laboratory and the clinic. Examples of these approaches are the elegant studies of Simmons and Russell on the lack of antigenicity of the rodent trophoblast[5] and the intriguing (if not yet fully explained) work on the abnormalities of immune regulation found in recurrent spontaneous abortion.[6] One should add to these approaches the careful observation of "experiments of nature" (to use Robert A. Good's felicitous phrase), such as occur with the transplacental passage of autoimmune antibodies.[7] Taken together with the more recent sophisticated methodologies of cellular immunology and molecular biology, these diverse pathways have provided considerable insight into a fascinating but difficult area of study.

To return to the paradox, it would be appropriate here to restate and modify the list of mechanisms Alan Beer and his colleagues provided in 1981 that might explain "the nonrejection of allogeneic fetoplacental implants."[8] One could consider this to be an update of the concept outlined in Medawar's "viviparity" paper of 28 years previously.

1. Complete separation of maternal and fetal blood circulations.
2. Afferent blockade in the feto-maternal complex, analogous to the concept of the uterus as an immunologically privileged site.
3. An immunologic barrier at the feto–maternal interface because of:
    a. failure to express paternal alloantigens, or
    b. masking of expressed paternal alloantigens.
4. Endocrinologically mediated local (decidual) inhibition of alloreactivity.
5. Production of immunosuppressive cells, antibodies, and/or factors, specific and/or nonspecific, by:
    a. fetus and b. mother

This book will attempt to explore each of these possibilities.

Finally, we should note that there is a new trend in thinking about the immunology of pregnancy. The older approach, exemplified in the above list, considers that maternal allograft mechanisms are potentially *harmful* to the fetus, and thus they must be overcome, bypassed, or subverted in order to achieve optimal pregnancy success. Within this context, the fetus is usually referred to as an *allograft*.

More recent concepts of the interrelation between immunologically competent cells and tissue growth factors are leading investigators to explore the idea that materno–fetal alloreactivity may be *beneficial* to fetal growth and survival. With this new thinking has come a tendency to reject the term *fetal allograft* and to redescribe the phenomenon of pregnancy as one of *"constructive symbiosis"*[7] or even *"programmed symbiosis"* (G. Chaouat, personal communication). These are intriguing neologisms, embodying intriguing new ideas. Although I shall often lapse and use the shorter term of "allograft," we should all realize that newer concepts are helping us to understand *the immunologic paradox of pregnancy.*

References

1. Medawar PB: Some immunological and endocrinological problems raised by the evolution of viviparity in vertebrates. *Symp Soc Exp Biol* 1953; 11: 320–338.
2. Billingham RE: Transplantation immunity and the maternal-fetal relation. *N Engl J Med* 1964; 270: 667–672.
3. Billingham RE: Transplantation immunity and the materno-fetal relation. *N Engl J Med* 1964; 270: 720–725.
4. Beer AE, Billingham RE: Immunobiology of mammalian reproduction, in Dixon FJ, Kunkel HG (eds): *Advances in Immunology.* New York, Academic Press; 1971: 1–84.
5. Simmons RL: Histoincompatibility and the survival of the fetus: Current controversies. *Transplant Proc* 1969; 1: 47–60.
6. Rocklin RE, Kitzmiller JL, Kaye MD: Immunobiology of the maternal-fetal relationship. *Ann Rev Med* 1979; 30: 375–404.
7. Scott JS: Pregnancy—nature's experimental system: Transient manifestations of immunological diseases in the child. *Lancet* 1976; i: 78–80.
8. Beer AE, Quebbeman JF, Ayers JWT, et al: Major histocompatibility complex antigens, maternal and paternal immune responses and chronic habitual abortions in humans. *Am J Obstet Gynecol* 1981; 141: 987–999.

Contents

Chapter 1

The Immune System

This chapter will present an outline of the structure and functions of the immune system. The approach will differ somewhat from others, as it will not be an exhaustive treatise on the immune system. Our knowledge of the immune system, although far from complete, is already so detailed that such a treatise would be inappropriate (and beyond the capability of this author). Besides, there are excellent comprehensive textbooks that serve this purpose well.[1-6] Instead, this chapter will present an overview of the immune system, emphasizing those facts and concepts that will be useful in understanding the material *in this book.*

The immune system is a large and complicated set of elements widely distributed in the body. Its primary "purpose" (if one thinks teleologically) appears to be to protect the organism from harmful foreign pathogens. To do this, it has developed an elaborate biochemical apparatus. This machinery must, of course, distinguish between those foreign pathogens to which it needs to react, and those very similar (but not identical) self components against which it should not react. Hence, the common view is that the function of the immune system is to distinguish "self" from "nonself." From this viewpoint, the outstanding concept of this book is the fact that *the fetus—uniquely—is both self and nonself.* How the immune system handles this unique situation is the main (but not the only) subject of this book.

Characteristics of the Immune System

The immune system has a number of interesting characteristics. None of them is unique to the system, but together they shed some light on the distinctive nature of the system as a whole.

Specificity

Immune responses are directed to specific antigenic determinants (often called epitopes). Immune recognition can distinguish between closely-related epitopes. The mechanism
responsible for this specificity is a series of receptors for antigen
that occur on T and B cells. The B cell type of specific molecule
(immunoglobulin) is present on B cells and also in soluble forms
as antibody, which can be measured in serum and secretions.
The T cell specific recognition molecule [the T cell receptor (TcR)]
exists on the surface of T cells, and rarely (if ever) in free secreted forms. The T cell receptor and immunoglobulin may be
considered to be the only immunologically specific elements in
the immune system.

A revolution in our conceptual basis for understanding the
immune system occurred at the end of the 1950s. *The clonal
selection theory* was put forth simultaneously by David Talmage
in the US and Macfarlane Burnet in Australia. Earlier theories
of the development of immunological specificity are usually
called "instructive" because it was believed that the foreign antigen came in and "instructed" the immune system to respond to it.
In terms of these theories, the immunological repertoire was the
mirror image of the repertoire of antigenic structures that had
been encountered. The clonal selection theory turned these
concepts upside down, by stating that *immunological specificity
developed during ontogeny prior to antigenic exposure.*
According to the new theory, the immune machinery was composed of sets (clones) of lymphocytes, each clone able to make
an antibody, but only to the particular foreign antigen that "fit"
that clone. The critical part of the theory was that these clones
differentiated randomly prior to the encounter with antigen.
Instead of instructing the system, the antigen merely selected the
appropriate preexisting clone whose surface immunoglobulin
molecule fitted it best. Other clones were unaffected. An important part of the theory was that clones that had the potential to
react against self antigens either did not develop or were purged

in some way. Of course, this aspect of immunology is crucial for our understanding of autoimmunity.

The clonal selection theory was hailed by some, but also ran into resistance. Critics claimed that such a system was:

1. *Too risky.* Suppose your random assortment of clones did not happen to contain one able to recognize, for example, diphtheria toxin?
2. *Too demanding.* Our genetic apparatus could not afford to commit so much of its precious DNA to the development of all the genes needed for all those clones.
3. *Too wasteful.* Why should the immune system expend all the energy and materials to develop clones of lymphocytes able to react with all sorts of antigens, including many we will probably never encounter (such as moon bugs)?

All of these (and other) criticisms to the contrary notwithstanding, the clonal selection theory has proven to be a brilliant and original insight, combining the best of both evolutionary and genetic biology. The fact that it was developed before T cells and their receptors were distinguished from B cells and immunoglobulins, and yet was perfectly suitable for both T and B systems, attests to the power and flexibility of the model.

Memory

After the immune system has encountered an antigen and responded to it, the system is changed. Usually, it has become "primed" by the first encounter, so that a second exposure to the same antigen leads to an augmented or *anamnestic* (remembered) response. This response is not only greater than the primary response but it is qualitatively different as well. This augmented and altered secondary response can be thought of as an example of "positive" immunologic memory. On occasion, however, the encounter with antigen leaves the immune system altered in a different way. Sometimes, the first exposure to the antigen (usually delivered in a special form or by a particular route) does *not* result in a measurable response, but also changes the system so that a subsequent exposure to the same antigen (in immunogenic form) fails to elicit the expected response. This phenomenon, called *acquired immunologic tolerance,* might be considered as an example of "negative" immunologic memory.

Mobility

The elements of the immune system are mobile. This includes lymphocytes, immunoglobulins, cytokines, and complement components, all of which move around the body. The consequences of this feature of the immune system are profound, yet obvious. For example, sensitization by a contact allergen on one part of the skin—because of the mobility of the stimulated clone of relevant T cells—leads to a state of systemic sensitization. Thus a later application of the same antigen will elicit a recall response anywhere on the body.

Replicability

The lymphocytic elements of the immune system can replicate, and ordinarily do so during immune responses. This capability endows the system with a means of amplifying its responses by increasing the number of responding elements. However, there are dangers here as well. There must be mechanisms to limit the expansion of clonal responses and to put a cap on cellular proliferation, lest the commitment to a particular set of stimuli interfere with other antigenically unrelated but equally important responses.

Cooperativity

It is now clear that an immune response involves interactions between a surprising variety of cells and molecules. This degree of cooperativity is a requirement for a system that is so diverse. The means by which macrophages, T cells, B cells, mast cells, cytokines, HLA molecules, complement proteins, and even other elements of the body are interlinked is one of the most active areas of immunological research.

Immunologic Machinery

Our knowledge of the elements of the immunologic machinery—the cells and molecules that make up the immune system—is growing extremely fast. The number and quality of immunological experiments and research projects, as well as immunological papers, reviews, books, and conferences continue to increase. This trend reflects not only our growing capabilities but the inherent complexity of the system that can only be compared with the complexity of the genetic apparatus and the nervous system. (In this context, it is amusing to look back at earlier, simpler days, when there was only one kind of lymphocyte, two antibody isotypes, one complement pathway, and no cytokines. The situation now is very different.)

T Cells

T lymphocytes are derived from stem cell precursors in the bone marrow. These "generic" stem cells do not seem to have any antigenic specificity or reactivity. They travel via the blood and land near the outer cortical edge of the thymus. There they are subject to a variety of stimuli that leads to a number of critical processes. There is a high rate of cellular proliferation of these immature thymocytes and many of the cells die. They encounter the host major histocompatibility (MHC) gene products on the surface of the thymic epithelial cells. During the proliferative waves, the cells begin to differentiate and mature. They progress through a series of stages where the cell surface markers change and where they acquire antigenic specificity. This specificity is achieved via the random somatic rearrangement of the genes coding for the T cell receptor.

    Before we turn to the development of T cells in the thymus, it would be useful to introduce the system by which cell surface markers and hence cell phenotypes are determined. In general this is done by staining cells with various monoclonal (occasionally polyclonal) antibodies that bind to cell surface molecules that are characteristic of certain cells (and not characteristic of others), or that bind to molecules present in certain stages of a cell's lifespan (and not in other stages, i.e., are differentiation antigens). These antibodies identify structures designated by the abbreviation, *CD,* which stands for *cluster of differentiation.* This abbreviation is followed by a number. Thus, T cells in general have the CD2 marker. In common parlance, the term CD2 is sometimes used for the molecule itself, but is also used to identify the antibody to that molecule, although it is more correct to speak of the reagent as anti-CD2. Sometimes the nature and/ or function of the molecule on the cell is known (the CD2 molecule is the receptor for sheep erythrocytes on human T cells) and sometimes it is not.

    The history of the use of these markers has been confusing, at least partly because there were a number of nomenclatures in which different identification symbols were used to designate the same reagent. For instance, the CD4 molecule on T cells was identified by both the Leu 3 antibody made by one company and by the OKT4 antibody made by another company. The current system of unambiguous CD designations has clarified the field.

    Table 1 outlines much of the commonly used CD terminology. These molecules and the corresponding reagents will be referred to throughout this book.

    Returning to the T cell, Fig. 1 shows a schema in which one can trace the development of thymocytes from immature, "generic" antigen-nonresponsive precursors to mature clones of antigen specific cells. During this time, the cells acquire and lose cell surface markers in a defined pattern. For instance, the common T cell marker, CD2, is acquired early in the differentiative pathway, and is retained. Then, the CD3 marker is displayed,

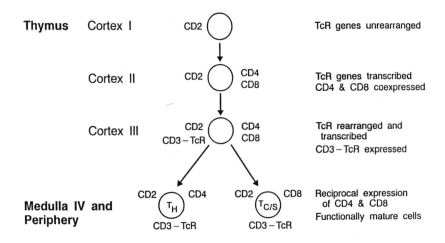

Fig. 1. Primitive pre-T cells arrive in the thymic cortex from the bone marrow. They soon develop CD2 (the sheep RBC receptor). As they move through the cortex, they express both CD4 and CD8 molecules, thus becoming "double positive" T cells. The TcR genes are rearranged and transcribed, and certain clones are purged by negative selection (not shown). The most mature cells in the cortex are "double positive" for CD4 and CD8 and have the CD3-T cell receptor (TcR) expressed. Further maturation involves loss of either CD4 or CD8 leading to cells in the periphery that are functionally mature. These cells are CD2+, CD3-TcR+ CD4+ ("helpers" = Th) and CD2+, CD3-TcR+ CD8+ ("cytotoxic/ suppressor" = Tc/s) cells.

and is also retained. (As we will see, this marker is intimately linked to the T cell receptor for antigen.) The CD4 and CD8 markers, which commonly are said to identify "T helper" and "T cytotoxic/suppressor" cells, respectively, appear nearly at the same time. Cells having both of these molecules are called "double positive" cells. Double positive cells later lose one or the other of these markers so that the progeny, as they exist as the most mature T cells in the thymus, and, after their exit, as typical mature T cells in the periphery, are "single positive." They carry either the CD4 or the CD8 markers but they do not carry both.

Table 1

Selected Cell Differentiation Antigens

(Where Corresponding Monoclonal Antibodies Are Useful in Cell Detection and Analysis)

Antigen	Some earlier designations	Distributions	Comments
CD2	T-11 Leu 5 LFA 2	All T, NK	Receptor for sheep rbc Accessory molecule for T APC interaction
CD3	T3, Leu 4	All mature T	Assoc. with TcR for antigen.
CD4	T4 Leu 3	50–70% mature T	Assoc. with class II HLA-restricted responses Often called a marker for "helper" T cells Receptor for HIV
CD8	T8 Leu 2	30–40% mature T	Assoc. with class I HLA-restricted responses Often called a marker for "cytotoxic/suppressor" T cells
CD11b	Leu 15 OKMI	Monos, NK Granulocytes Some T	Reciprocal with CD4 Part of complement receptor #3 Assoc. with CD 18

CD16	Leu 11	NK Granulocytes	FcγR III
CD19,20	B4 B1	B	
CD21	B2	B Dendritic cells	Complement receptor #2 EBV receptor
CD25	Tac	Activated T Some B, NK	Part of IL-2R
CD29	4B4	SomeCD4+ and CD8+	"Memory" T cell marker Reciprocal with CD45 RA
CD32	2E1	B, monocytes Granulocytes Platelets	FcγR II
CD35		All B, a few T Monocytes Granulocytes	Complement receptor #1
CD45 RA	2H4	Some CD4+ Some CD8+ Some B, monos	"Naive" T cell marker Reciprocal with CD45 RO
CD45 RO	UCHL1	Some CD4+ Some CD8+	"Memory" T cell marker (3bR)
CD46		Leukocytes Epithelial cells Fibroblasts Trophoblasts	Membrane cofactor protein (MCP) complement regulation A TLX antigen?
CD56	Leu-19	NK cells	
CD57	Leu -7	NK cells	
	HNK-1	Some T cells	

Specific reactivity for the T cell resides in the structure of the T cell receptor (TcR). This complex molecule is derived from a number of genes belonging to the immunoglobulin super-gene family, through a series of complicated gene rearrangements.[7] The result is a dictionary of different TcRs, each "word" of which is expressed on a small group of T cells that then constitute a *clone*. The members of the most common family of TcRs are each composed of two membrane-bound polypeptide chains, called α and β. Each of these is polymorphic, and the individual specificity of a given TcR depends on the "fit" of the appropriate antigen into the cavity formed by the variable regions of the α and β chains most distant from the cell surface. The analogy of the α,β chain structure of the TcR to the heavy-light chain structure of immunoglobulin molecules should be obvious. Indeed, the α and β chains of the TcR belong to the immunoglobulin gene superfamily.[8,9] The TcR is physically linked to the CD3 complex. Therefore, the identification of a T cell bearing CD3 is generally felt to identify a mature T cell belonging to some antigen-specific clone or other. Conversely, a cell with some characteristics of T cells but without CD3 would be considered to be a cell that is not clonally restricted and therefore not reactive to specific antigen. In humans, attention is paid not only to the number of T cells of various types, but to their relative frequencies, i.e., their ratios. The most famous of these is the ratio of "T helpers" to "T suppressors." This Th/Ts ratio is normally greater than one in human peripheral blood. It is greatly lessened or "inverted" during the course of AIDS infection. At least in part, this is because the HIV virus infects the lymphocyte by binding to the CD4 molecule on Th cells, thus leading to Th cell destruction. The Th/Ts ratio does have practical value in AIDS medicine, but it is not specific for the HIV virus.

Recently, a new class of T cell receptor was recognized, called the γδ TcR. This receptor is similar to the αβ T cell receptor in that it has two polymorphic transmembrane polypeptide chains that may be disulfide-linked or noncovalently attached to each other. These are termed γ and δ chains. γδ T cells express the CD3 complex but not the α and β chains of the TcR. Their function is unknown, but they are enriched in immature thymus populations and in epithelial tissue.[10]

T cells serve a large number of purposes in the immune system, and so have been called "the master cells" of immunology. They are responsible not only for allograft recognition and rejection but for defense against intracellular parasites, for antiviral protection (when the virus is cell-associated), for delayed hypersensitivity reactions, and for helping B cells make antibody. Many people believe that in autoimmune conditions, whether the effector mechanism is T cell or B cell, an abnormal T cell is at fault. Furthermore, active downregulation of immune processes can be carried out by T cells with specific or nonspecific downregulating activities. These are called suppressor T cells (Ts) and are described briefly later in this chapter.

B Cells

B cells also develop from stem cell precursors in the yolk sac and fetal liver, and later in the bone marrow itself. They progress through a series of maturation stages, during which they, like T cells, display a variety of cell markers. From the standpoint of this book, it is the immunoglobulin genes and gene products that are most important. B cell precursors develop their specific immunological reactivity via a series of random somatic gene segment rearrangements of genes that are also members of the immunoglobulin gene superfamily. This process culminates in the creation of another "library" of specific antigen receptors different from, but related to, the TcR. These receptors exist as a complex of the variable regions of the heavy (H) and light (L) chains on the Fab (Fraction that is antigen-binding) region of the immunoglobulin molecule (Fig. 2). Thus, B cell development results in a set of clones, each of which has a specific immunoglobulin (Ig) expressed, able to react with one antigen that fits it best (or with a structurally similar, crossreacting antigen). The

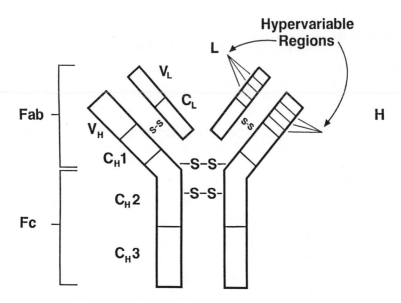

Fig. 2. Prototype of immunoglobulin molecule showing heavy (H) and light (L) chains, each with common (C) and variable (V) regions and each with hypervariable regions. Antigen combines with antibody in cavity formed by hypervariable end of H and L chains. These two chains are joined by disulfide bonds (S–S). Light chains have one variable (V_L) and one constant (C_L) region. Heavy chains have one variable (V_H) and three or four common regions (C_H1 through 3 or C_H1 through 4). Light chains and V_H and C_H1 make up fragments for antigen-binding (Fab) region. Other common regions of the H chain make up fragments that crystalize (Fc) region. The COOH ends of the molecules are in the constant regions and the NH_2 ends of the molecules are in the variable regions.

variable region of the Ig is attached to a constant region that is characteristic for a given Ig isotype. The constant region is part of the Fc (Fraction that crystallizes or is constant) part of the Ig molecule. As shown in Fig. 3, B cells progress through stages where IgM is the first isotype expressed, initially in the cytoplasm and later on the cell surface. As immune development continues, and antigen stimulation occurs, B cells *switch* their con-

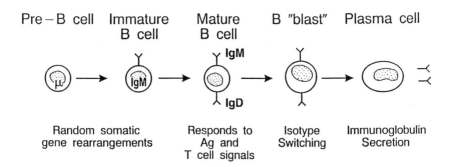

Fig. 3. B cells mature mainly in the bone marrow. Pre-B cells only express μ chains in the cytoplasm. Immature B cells express IgM in the cytoplasm and on the cell surface. Mature B cells express IgM and IgD. When driven by antigen and appropriate T cell signals, mature B cells undergo isotype switching and evolve into immunoglobulin secreting plasma cells.

stant region expression, so that a variety of immunoglobulin isotypes, e.g., IgM, IgG, IgA, IgD, and IgE are expressed and secreted. The final stage of B cell development is the mature plasma cell, able to secrete immunoglobulins.

Macrophages

Macrophages are mature members of the mononuclear phagocyte cell family. They are not related to lymphocytes, and they have no antigenic specificity. They are important in the context of this book in two ways. First, macrophages (and the related set of cells called *dendritic cells*) are essential for the presentation of antigen to antigen-reactive cells. T cells, for instance, are not capable of recognizing and reacting to antigenic material unless it is "presented through the right diplomatic pathways." This presentation involves at least two processes; the breaking down of complex antigens to more palatable simpler epitopes and the display of these epitopes in the right configuration on the macrophage surface. This latter generally means that the "nominal antigen" or epitope is presented to the clonally-selected antigen-reactive cell *in the context of a component of the major histocompatibility complex.* In other words, lymphocytes, particularly T lymphocytes, do not recognize and react to "free" antigen, but to antigen-MHC. Macrophages have both class I and class II MHC on their surface, and they can biochemically "process" complex antigens. For these reasons macrophages are, not surprisingly, efficient antigen-presenting cells. Second, macrophages are also important components of antimicrobial and inflammatory processes.

Cytokines

Cytokines are soluble molecules that are crucial for the development and function of the immune system, but are not peculiar to it. Indeed, they provide important links between immune and nonimmune processes, such as hematopoiesis. Cytokines include the interferons, the interleukins, and a number of growth factors and molecules such as tumor necrosis factors (TNFs). The list of cytokines has grown explosively, and a number of them and their receptors have been cloned and sequenced. In addition, monoclonal antibodies to the cytokines and their receptors are now available for almost all cytokines. Research in these fields is very active, and this section will just be able to outline the salient features of the subject.

Cytokines have a number of common properties, although they belong to chemically different families. They are small polypeptides that are produced by a variety of cells and are able to act on a variety of cells. In fact, one cytokine can be produced by more than one cell and can act on more than one target. For example, interleukin-1 (IL-1) can be produced by macrophages as well as keratinocytes. IL-1 can act on fibroblasts, lymphocytes, hepatocytes, and other cells. Table 2 lists the best-studied cytokines and points out their molecular weights, primary cells of origin, and primary targets. More detailed information is available elsewhere.[11,12]

Cytokines probably can act at a distance, but have very low concentrations in the blood and body fluids and very short half-lives. Therefore they are most efficient acting in *paracrine* fashion, i.e., on neighboring cells. They can also act in *autocrine* fashion, i.e., on the very cell that produces it.

Cytokines generally produce their effects via binding to a specific receptor on the target cell. The cytokine may, in part, be responsible for upregulating that receptor, as happens with IL-2. The cytokine receptors may be present on a variety of target cells, accounting for the diversity of effects of even a single cytokine. Similarly, a cell may have receptors for more than one cytokine, accounting for what has been called the *degeneracy* of cytokine specificity. To put it another way, one cannot deduce the presence of a specific cytokine from some effect on a target cell—that effect may have been produced by one or another cytokine. Recently, cytokines have been shown to act synergistically, and the order of cytokine presentation to a given target cell can be critical in determining the final signal.

Cytokines can act in positive and negative ways and can positively and negatively regulate each other.

Interleukins comprise a loose group of molecules that, properly speaking, should provide signals only between leukocytes. Interleukins, as well as other cytokines, are pleomorphic in their activities and are not limited to leukocytes in terms of their origin or destination. As can be seen, interleukins can be produced by a variety of cells, and they overlap in their effector functions. There are a number of functional groupings that can be made.

IL-1, IL-6, and IL-8 are proinflammatory. IL-2 and IL-9 are important for lymphocyte proliferation. IL-4 and IL-5 are critical for immunoglobulin isotype switching, IL-4 controlling IgE production and IL-5 being involved in IgA production. IL-10 may not be properly termed an interleukin, but it has the interesting capability of limiting interleukin production, providing a needed negative feedback mechanism.

Table 2
Cytokines

	Structure	Made by	Actions
Interleukin-1 (IL-1)	2 forms (α,β) 18 kDa	Macrophages Keratinocytes	Pro-inflammatory endogenous pyrogen lymphoid cofactor fibroblast activator hepatocyte stimulator (→ acute phase proteins)
Interleukin-2 (IL-2)	15 kDa	Many T cells	T cell growth B cell growth factor NK cell growth factor
Interleukin-3 (IL-3)	23 kDa	T cells Mast cells	Multi-CSF (a hematopoietic [GF]) Mast cell proliferation
Interleukin-4 (IL-4)	20 kDa	T cells Mast cells B cells	B cell growth and differentiation B cell isotype switching to IgE Class II MHC induction on cell surfaces
Interleukin-5 (IL-5)	50 kDa	T cells Mast cells B cells?	Eosinophil growth and differentiation IgA synthesis
Interleukin-6 (IL-6)	26 kDa	Macophages T cells Fibroblasts	B cell differentiation Hepatocyte stimulator (→ acute phase proteins) Plasma cell growth
Interleukin-7 (IL-7)	25 kDa		Proliferation of pre-B, thymocytes T cells

Interleukin-8 (IL-8)	6-10 kDa Member of multigene family, incl. PF4, β-thrombo-globulin	Keratinocytes Fibroblasts Monocytes	Neutrophil chemotaxis and activation
Interleukin-9 (IL-9)	40 kDa	T cells	Proliferation of thymocytes and mast cells
Interleukin-10 (IL-10)	35 kDa	Th$_2$ Mastcells B cells?	Inhibits production of cytokines, e.g., IL1, IL-6, TNFα Enhances mast cell survival
Interferon-γ (IFNγ)	35 kDa	T cells: Th$_1$ CD8	Inhibits viral proliferation Inhibits IL-4 activity Activates macrophages Induces class II MHC
Tumor Necrosis (TNF)	2 forms: α β (lymphotoxin)	Macrophages Keratinocytesi T cells	Cytotoxic for virus-factor infected cells Cachexia and fever Macrophage and granulocyte activation and chemotaxis
Granulocyte-monocyte colony-stimulating factor (GM-CSF)	22 kd	T cells Keratinocytes Hematopobtic stoma	Hematopoietic growth factor for monocytes and granulocytes
Transforming Growth Factor β (TGFβ)	Several forms Inactive precursor	Megakaryocytes Chondrocytes	Angiogenic Inhibits endothelium B cell stimulation Wound healing

Interferons comprise a set of cytokines that were first identified because of their ability to interfere with the superinfection of cells by certain viruses. There are 3 major classes of interferons (IFNs)—α, β, and γ. Leukocytes make IFN-α and both fibroblasts and epithelial cells make IFN-β. IFN-γ is of greatest interest to the immunologist. It is made primarily by activated CD8$^+$ cells. It has a number of activities, among which are the ability to activate macrophages and to upregulate the level of class I and II MHC molecules on the cell surface.

Other cytokines are immunologically pertinent. Hematopoietic cell differentiation is controlled by *colony-stimulating factors* (CSFs) and a number of these are made by lymphoid cells, including G-CSF (granulocyte-CSF) and GM-CSF (granulocyte-monocyte CSF). These pathways provide connections between the immune and the hematopoietic systems. Still other cytokines such as tumor necrosis factors (TNF α and β) and transforming growth factor β (TGF-β) are important in inflammation, tumor cell control, and cell growth regulation.[13]

Immunoglobulins

The immunoglobulin family of molecules consists of 5 members, IgG, IgA, IgM, IgD, IgE. These 5 isotypes are distinguished by the possession of unique heavy chain constant regions, namely γ, α, μ, δ, and ε. There are subclasses of IgG, namely IgG1, IgG2, IgG3, and IgG4, and of IgA, namely IgA1 and IgA2. Each Ig molecule consists of heavy chains of the appropriate isotype, and either kappa (κ) or lambda (λ) light chains. Table 3 gives some basic properties of the major immunoglobulin classes and Fig. 2 gives the basic structure of a primitive Ig molecule. The unique structure of the immunoglobulin molecule made by a given clone of B cells resides in the unique three-dimensional cavity between the variable parts of the heavy chain (V_H) and the light chain (V_L). These in turn are determined by the amino acid sequences in these variable segments, particularly in the special hypervariable regions. This amino acid variability from one Ig molecules to another is, in turn, determined by a complex system of gene fragment rearrangements and mutations occurring at the DNA level during B cell development.[14,15] Owing to the differing biologic properties of the various heavy chains, each Ig isotype has different biological properties. As mentioned above, immunoglobulins are made by B cells and the membrane-bound Ig on the surface of a B cell should be considered as a sample of the kind of immunoglobulin the clonally selected B cell will make when appropriately stimulated by the cognate antigen, again, "when presented through the right diplomatic pathways." B cells are present throughout the entire body, in lymphoid organs, in mucosal tissues, and in the blood and lymph. The different immunoglobulin isotypes have differing relative and absolute concentrations in different tissues, and different half-lives in the blood and tissues. They play an important role in antimicrobial defense, but they also may comprise a major effector arm of autoimmune syndromes.

Idiotypes and anti-idiotypic antibodies.[16] In modern immunologic terminology, the unique antigen-binding portion of the Fab part of the Ig molecule that binds to the nominal antigen is called the *idiotope*, and the molecule bearing that unique structure is called an idiotype or *idiotypic antibody.* It is also called (for reasons that will be clearer in a moment) *"antibody-1."* Each antibody able to bind to a specific antigen has a unique three-dimensional configuration of that antigen-binding combination of heavy and light chain (idiotype). This configuration is subtly different from the corresponding part of another antibody molecule that recognizes a different antigen. Thus, we now have *three* huge families of receptors. Not only do we have a dictionary of T cell receptor "words" in the TcR dictionary, and we also have another lexicon of immunoglobulin Fab fragment "words" for the B cell clonal repertoire, but there can be a third dictionary of receptors on immunoglobulin molecules, designed to recognize the "words" in the B cell lexicon. These "anti-words" are called *anti-idiotypic antibodies.* It is a fact that in

Table 3
Human Immunoglobulins

	Mean adult serum concentration mg/dL ± SD	Complement fixation*	Placental transfer	Sedimentation constant, s	Half-life, d
Total IgG	1150 ± 300				
IgG$_1$	615 ± 200	++	Yes	7	21
IgG$_2$	295 ± 180	+	Yes	7	20
IgG$_3$	35 ± 14	+++	Yes	7	7
IgG$_4$	18 ± 16	0	Yes	7	21
IgM	100 ± 25	+++	No	19	10
IgA	200 ± 60	0	No	7	6
Surface IgA (secretory)	5			11	
IgD	3	0	No	7	3
IgE	0.005	0	No	8	2

*=None
+=Weak
++=Intermediate
+++=Strong

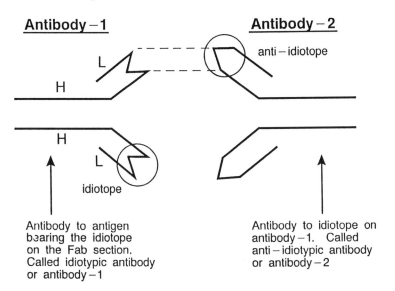

Antibody – 1

Antibody – 2

Antibody to antigen bearing the idiotope on the Fab section. Called idiotypic antibody or antibody – 1

Antibody to idiotope on antibody – 1. Called anti – idiotypic antibody or antibody – 2

Fig. 4. The antibody complementary to the antigen is antibody-1. It bears the idiotope for the antigen at the distal end of the Fab region, where the antigen fits into the cleft between the ends of the heavy (H) and light (L) chains. An antibody to that idiotope on antibody-1 is called antibody-2 or the anti-idiotypic antibody. Its distal Fab region is complementary to the idiotope on antibody-1.

experimental and naturally occurring conditions in humans and animals, the *production* of "ordinary" antibodies in a response to antigen can lead in turn to the production of anti-idiotypic antibodies. These anti-antibodies or antibody-2 molecules are complementary to and bind to the first antibodies. As one might expect in this game of mirror images, antibody-2 may resemble the original antigen although this is not necessarily so. Figure 4 gives a schematic presentation of how antigen antibody-1 and antibody-2 might be related. In this example, the anti-idiotypic antibody resembles the original triangular antigen.

As there are structural and functional resemblances between T cell receptors and immunoglobulins, there is no reason why one might not develop a T cell with its receptor complementary to the TcR of another T cell. This could function as an idiotype-

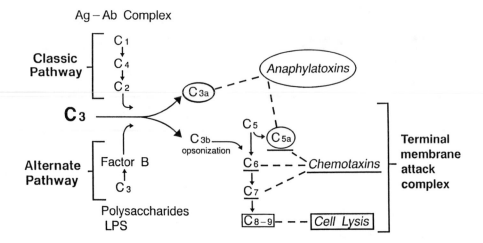

Fig. 5. The two complement pathways, the classic and the alternate each can activate C3, which is thus the central complement molecule. Activation of C3 by either pathway leads to activation of C5-9, the terminal components. During terminal component activation, products are generated which lead to mediator release (anaphylatoxins), chemotasix, and cell lysis.

anti-idiotype pair, where the TcR complementary to the peptide-MHC complex is TcR-1 (idiotype) and the second T cell responding to the idiotype is TcR-2 (anti-idiotype).

Complement

The complement system is very complex, and it is difficult to deal with it in abbreviated fashion. Either one says too little about it or one goes into such detail that the reader is lost in a maze of enzymatic twistings. In essence, it consists of a large group of proteins that functionally comprise two interacting and overlapping pathways. Figure 5 shows a basic outline of these pathways.

At the top is the *classical complement pathway,* which begins with the activation of C1 and goes to C3. Below is the *alternate complement pathway*, which begins with the activation of C3 and factor B. Thus both initial activation steps in complement metabolism meet at C3 activation. The terminal steps of both pathways go from C3 to C9 and are identical. The proteins in the pathways function as enzymes, each acting on the subsequent protein and converting it from an inactive to an active form. In many ways, the complement cascades resemble blood coagulation cascades. There are also many feedback mechanisms involved, which keep the complement systems modulated.

In general, the two pathways are set in motion by different means. The classical pathway is typically activated by antigen–antibody complexes and by aggregated immunoglobulins of the IgG or IgM isotypes. The alternate pathway responds to IgA complexes and to some polysaccharides, such as lipopolysaccharide or dextran, even in the absence of antibody. There are important biological consequences of complement activation. As many of these involve activation of C3 and the components further down the cascade, they can be seen when either the classical or the alternate pathway is activated. The activation of complement and the enzymatic action of the complement components release fragments of complement proteins. Some of these have biologic properties that are not possessed by the native uncleaved proteins. For instance, the cleaved component of C3, namely C3a, and the cleaved component of C5, called C5a, are powerful chemoattractants for polymorphonuclear (PMN) leukocytes, and thus complement activation can be a major instigator of inflammatory reactions. C3b is an important mediator of opsonization, as molecules with C3b on their surfaces are quickly taken up by the various phagocytic systems that include cells with receptors for C3b, namely macrophages and PMNs. Complement is also important in solubilizing and removing immune complexes.

The activation of the terminal sequences of the complement cascade leads to the "membrane attack complex." This mechanism provides a means to lyse target cells, such as gram negative bacteria. On occasion, it can lead to intravascular hemolysis if the target cell is an erythrocyte coated with IgM or IgG. Con-

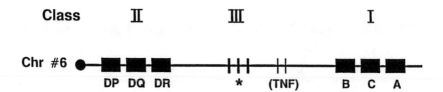

Fig. 6. The genes for MHC are on human chromosome #6. Closest to the centromere are the class II genes. Class III genes (*) include complement components C2 and C4. Between them and the class I genes are the loci encoding TNF.

versely, the ability of antibody to "fix" (use up) complement in vitro is the basis for several old but sensitive immunoassays called complement fixation tests.

The Major Histocompatibility Complex (MHC) and HLA Antigens

The function of the immune system is intimately connected with the system of histocompatibility or "transplantation" antigens. The predominant area of interest is the major histocompatibility complex (MHC) whose genes are found on the 6th chromosome in humans. (The terminology implies the existence of other, minor histocompatibility genes, but they will not be discussed here.) The MHC in humans is called the human leukocyte antigen (HLA) complex, because the antigens were first discovered using circulating leukocytes. We know now that HLA antigens are found on virtually all the nucleated cells in the body, but the term, HLA, has remained. The topology of this gene complex is shown in Fig. 6. HLA genes A, B, and C are called class I MHC, whereas genes in the DR, DP, and DQ are called class II genes. The genes and gene products in the class I category resemble those in the class II group and the two systems undoubtedly arose by gene duplication. Between them are genes for some of the complement components in each of the comple-

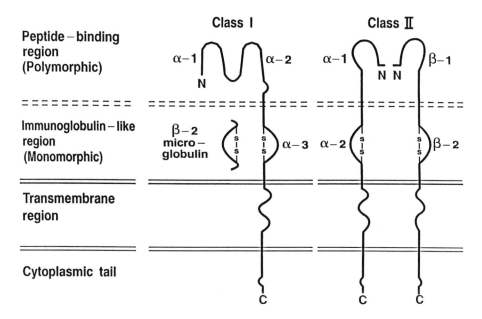

Fig. 7. MHC molecules each contain an α and α β chain. Class I molecules have an a chain with 3 domains, where the cytoplasmic tail is the C-terminal end. Class I molecules use β-2 microglobulin as the β chain. Class II molecules have α and β chains, each of which has the C-terminal end of the cytoplasm. The antigen-binding (polymorphic) ends of the class I and class II molecules are the N-terminal portions, which are structurally the most distant from the cell membrane.

ment pathways. Although they do not function as transplantation antigens, they are parts of the immune system and do show limited polymorphisms. Also included in this broad region are the genes for TNF, although it is not clear why they occur within the part of the chromosome containing the MHC.

The basic structures of typical class I molecule and typical class II molecules are shown in Fig. 7. Each molecule has two polypeptide chains. Class I has an α chain that has two regions, α-1 and α-2, which are polymorphic and are located away from the cell surface, and a nonpolymorphic constant region, α-3, nearer the cell surface. This end of the molecule is anchored in the membrane by a transmembrane section that ends in a χ-terminal tail in the cytoplasm. This basic structure itself suggests that "outside" signals can be transmitted by the free end of the molecule to the "inside" cellular machinery. Class I molecules have as their second chain the β-2 microglobulin ($\beta_2 m$) molecule that is not polymorphic. Class II molecules each have an α and $\alpha\beta$ chain, and each of these has the same basic configuration as does the α chain of class I. The astute reader will notice the similarities in the basic molecular structures of the class I and class II molecules on the one hand, and the immunoglobulin molecules on the other hand—two polypeptide chains with constant regions anchored in the cell membrane and polymorphic regions further outside the cell. (There are even more similarities in the internal structure of each chain, such as the location of intrachain disulfide bridges.) Thus it is no surprise to find that the genes for HLA class I and II molecules as well as the genes for immunoglobulin molecules all belong to the immunoglobulin gene superfamily.[17]

The immunologic reactions to HLA molecules are responsible for allograft rejection. There is polymorphism for each of the chains in the HLA complex (except $\beta_2 m$). There are approximately 24 alleles at the HLA A locus, and 50, 11, 18, 9, and 6 alleles at the HLA B, C, DR, DP, and DQ loci, respectively. The gene products for each allele are expressed codominantly on virtually every diploid nucleated cell in the body. (Erythrocytes, for example, do not expresses MHC products in humans.) Thus a cell will bear two HLA A gene products, one from one of the two maternal genes for HLA and one from one of the two paternal genes for HLA This arrangement is diagrammed in Fig. 8. In HLA terminology, the set of linked HLA genes and gene products inherited from one parent is called a *haplotype*. Thus, the mother in Fig. 8 has two haplotypes—HLA-A-1, B-5, DR-3 and HLA-A-2, B-8, DR-4. Two people sharing one haplotype with each other are *haploidentical;* if a person has two haplotypes both of which are also possessed by another person, these two are

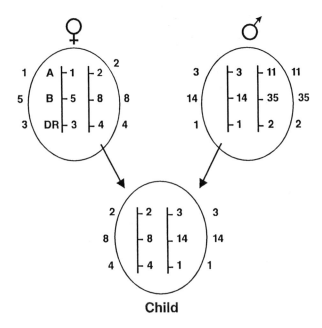

Child

Fig. 8. HLA gene products are codominantly expressed on the cell surface of most nucleated cells. In this example, the mother is HLA-A3,11, B14,35, DR1,2. The child inherits one chromosome #6 from each parent. It thus derives HLA-A2, B8, DR4 from the mother and HLA-A3, B14, DR1 from the father.

HLA-identical. Thus the child in Fig. 8 is haploidentical with the mother (via possession of HLA-A-2, B-8, DR-4) and haploidentical with the father by virtue of HLA-A-3, B-14, DR-1.

Immunologic Processes

Antigen Presentation

The immune system is bombarded by a constant stream of complex antigenic materials. One of the first jobs of the body is to make these antigens accessible, and this is done by a set of cells that are collectively known as "antigen-presenting" cells

(APCs). The typical APC is a macrophage, or a relative of the macrophage, the dendritic cell. These cells have a substantial internal machinery for engulfing, digesting, and representing antigenic determinants (epitopes) on their cell membranes so that they are "seen" (i.e., immunologically recognized) by the proper antigen-receptor, be it a TcR or an immunoglobulin. Furthermore, the APC must have the means to display the epitope in the correct configuration, and often, together with the correct class I or class II molecule. This is part of the MHC-restricted nature of immune responses *(see below)*. As macrophages are ubiquitous, antigen presentation can occur almost anywhere. However, other nonmacrophage type cells are also capable of presenting antigen. This includes B cells, activated endothelium, and even fibroblasts, under certain circumstances.[18]

There are two general pathways for the presentation of antigens.[19] Antigens to be recognized in the context of MHC class I are derived from the cytoplasm of the APC. For example, a virus is degraded by the APC and viral peptides are present within the cell before being transported to the surface class I molecules. By contrast, antigens to be presented by MHC class II are endocytosed by the APC and then are degraded in endosomes before surface presentation together with class II. This would be the fate of complex proteins, for instance.

T Cell Processes

T Cell Recognition and MHC Restriction

T cells in general do not recognize "free" antigen. In order for T cell activation to occur, the T cell receptor must be engaged by a complex consisting of both the epitope best fitting the groove in the TcR as well as an MHC molecule, either class I or class II. (Recognition of alloantigens is a special case, discussed below). The development of the T cell dictionary in the thymus has resulted in TcRs able to recognize epitopes in the context of the person's own MHC. This is called *MHC restriction,* and it implies that a

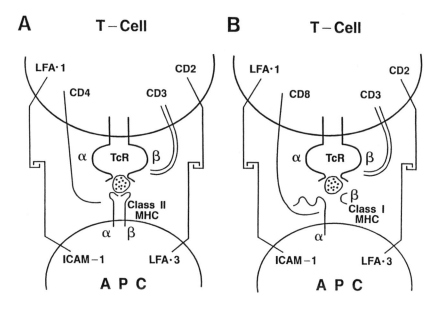

Fig.9. T cell-MHC interactions. A CD4 ("helper") T cell (A, left) has a TcR which interacts with antigen (stippled) which is associated with MHC class II on the antigen-presenting cell (APC). The APC may be a macrophage, or B cell, or other cell. The TcR is stabilized by CD3. Accessory molecules such as LFA-1 and CD2 on the T cell interact with ICAM-1 and LFA-3 on the APC.A CD8 ("cytotoxic/suppressor") T cell (B, right), has its TcR interact with antigen (stippled) which is associated with MHC class I on the APC.

person's T cell will not respond to even the "correct" epitope unless it is presented with the person's own MHC (or a genetically identical MHC from someone else.) Furthermore, different types of T cells require different types of MHC on the antigen-presenting cell. CD4$^+$ T cells respond to antigen in the context of MHC class II and CD8$^+$ T cells respond to antigen in the context of MHC class I. This is diagrammed in Fig. 9.

Recognition of Alloantigens

Recognition of alloantigens shows a variation on the above theme. An alloantigen functions as both the epitope and as MHC, in this case a foreign MHC. This complex is recognized by a T cell, and many immunologists consider that foreign MHC antigens resemble the complex of a nominal epitope plus a self MHC molecule. In this sense, recognition of, and response to an alloantigen could be considered a "crossreaction," i.e., a situation where a T cell clone could recognize either of two almost identical moieties—a nominal foreign epitope-plus-self-MHC or an alloantigen that fortuitously looks just like it. It must be remembered that the T cell system includes a series of fairly large clones of alloreactive cells.

Activation and Proliferation Patterns

In general, T cells exist in the nondividing(G-O) state. Triggering them by engaging the right cell surface structure sets in motion a series of biochemical changes that may lead to a variety of processes, including cell division, a change in the state of differentiation and the expression of differentiation markers, the start of or an alteration in the kinds and amounts of cytokine production or the expression of an effector function.

Upon meeting the proper stimulus, a resting T cell has signals induced at its surface membrane. These processes include various calcium-dependent pathways involving protein kinases and phospholipases. In turn, there is nuclear activation of genes encoding cytokines and cytokine receptors, such as IL-2 and IL-2R. This results in protein synthesis, "blast transformation" and ultimately cell division. At the same time, other cytokines can be produced (Table 2) that can act in autocrine fashion on the T cells themselves or in paracrine fashion on neighboring T cells, B cells, and macrophages.

From the population standpoint, one may discern three patterns of T cell activation: clonal expansion, superantigen activation, and mitogen stimulation. The results of these stimulatory activities are often measured by assessing T cell proliferation, but they can also be quantitated by examining intracellular events that are not necessarily linked to mitosis.

Clonal expansion is the activation of a clone of T cells by presenting to the TcR the appropriate foreign antigen in the context of the appropriate MHC molecule. Superantigen activation has only recently been described.[20] It involves the direct stimulation of a subset of T cell clones that bear one of the many families of TcRs that each share a common structure in the V_β chain of the TcR. The main source of superantigens is microbial flora, and different superantigens each stimulate different V_β families. These antigens and the responses to them may have a significant role in the etiology and pathogenesis of autoimmune diseases. Both clonal expansion and superantigen activation take place through engagement of sections of the T cell receptor. Mitogen stimulation, on the other hand, refers to the results of stimulating T cells via other structures that have nothing in common with the TcR. Thus, the mitogens will activate many (if not all) of the T cells regardless of their clonal commitment. The best studied mitogens are phytohemagglutinin (PHA) and Concanavalin A (Con A). Nonspecific (global) T cell activation can also be carried out by crosslinking the CD3 molecule via the use of insoluble anti-CD3.

Mixed Leukocyte Reactions (MLR)

Mixed leukocyte reactions (MLRs) occur when T cells of one MHC genotype are confronted by alloantigens of another genotype. MLRs are generally governed by differences at the class II locus, where the stimulator cell presents HLA DR to a T cell population from someone who does not possess that DR specificity. When this happens, the T cells become activated, and often divide. The extent of such activation can be measured by the incorporation of tritiated thymidine (a measure of DNA synthesis) or by IL-2 production, which is an intimate factor in T cell proliferation. In practice, there are "two-way" and "one-way" MLRs, and they are usually performed with the mononuclear leukocytes (which include monocytes, T, and B cells) of the peripheral blood. These will be referred to as peripheral blood leukocytes (PBL). A two-way MLR is set up by mixing PBL from two people and measuring cell activation, usually at the end of 5–7 days. If the people differ with regard to class II MHC, the result can be that person A's T cells can react to person B's HLA while person B's T cells are reacting to the HLA on the monocytes of person A. It is not possible to distinguish the contribution of the A anti-B reaction from the B anti-A reaction. Therefore, MLRs are usually done in a "one-way" manner. The PBL from one person (the stimulator) are inactivated in some way (usually by irradiation) prior to culturing so that the T cells in that population will not respond, but the monocytes will still be able to stimulate the T cells of the other person (the responder).

As mentioned, the T cell repertoire includes a substantial number of clones of alloreactive cells able to mount an MLR against foreign MHC class II bearing cells that have never been encountered. Such an MLR, when it is performed, might be considered to be a "primary" MLR. In considering transplantation reactions, one might want to know if the MLR might be "rigged" to demonstrate *allograft memory,* that is, to show that a person has encountered and reacted to the MHC class II in the past. In that case, one would expect that the clone(s) of T cells would have been expanded following the previous allograft reaction, so that there would be a faster, stronger MLR to the representation of the alloantigens. Not much work has been done in humans in this respect, but such *secondary MLR* reactions can be demonstrated by carefully controlling the number of reacting T cells and harvesting at an earlier time.

Autologous Mixed Leukocyte Reactions (AMLR)

The preceding discussion implies that there will be no MLR if a person's own responding T cells are cultured with his or her stimulator cells, because the two sets of cells are HLA-identical. However, small amounts of T cell proliferation can occur if the cultures are done in special ways. This is called an autologous mixed leukocyte reaction (AMLR). The reaction seems to involve a recognition of self-DR, as it is inhibited by anti-HLA-DR antiserum. The subject is controversial, but it has obvious relevance to self-reactivity and autoimmunity.[21]

T Cell Regulatory Mechanisms— "Help" and Suppression

It is now abundantly clear that immunological responses are closely regulated by positive and negative processes. The first demonstration of this concept occurred in my laboratory in 1966 where we showed that optimal antibody production required the interaction of two kinds of lymphoid cells, one coming from the thymus and the other coming from the bone marrow. We guessed, and J. F. A. P. Miller proved, that the bone marrow cells made the antibody while the thymus-derived cells "helped" in some as yet obscure way. For obvious reasons, these two sets of cells were called B and T cells, respectively, and the T cells were called "T helper cells" because of their role in augmenting B cell immunoglobulin production.

Our understanding of the cellular basis for T cell help was greatly aided by two discoveries, namely the identification of specific cell surface markers for various functional subsets of T cells, and the elucidation of various patterns of cytokine production by subclasses of T cells. There are still many aspects of these areas of study that are incompletely understood, but a safe simplification is that most "helper" T cells bear the CD4 marker and secrete IL-4, IL-5, and IL-6. These cytokines are B cell growth and differentiation factors and are essential for B cell clonal expansion and immunoglobulin isotype switching. These two functions in fact constitute the T cell "help" for B cells.

In 1970, Richard Gershon showed that T cells can also suppress B cell function and antibody synthesis. Thus emerged the first integrated concept of immune regulation. In terms of antibody production, the "net" observable result represents the balance between T cell help and T cell suppression. Later it was shown that most T cells that carry out suppressor activity bear the CD8 surface marker. In terms of mechanism, however, it has been difficult to determine just how T suppressor cells exert their down-regulatory functions. Some investigators have proudly denied the existence of suppressor T cells because of specific gene product or metabolic pathway could not be found. For the many immunologists who have found it simple to demonstrate T suppressor activity, the problem lies not in the existence of these cells and their effects but in the long-awaited demonstration of how they work. [22]

The concept of T cell control is central to the concept of immunoregulation. Thus T helpers (CD4) for CD8$^+$ T cytotoxic cells have been shown. There are obvious analogies between help and suppression in the T cell system and positive and negative (anti-idiotypic) pathways in B cell systems.

Cytotoxic Cells and Mechanisms

A prime means of immunologic control is exercised via cytotoxicity in which (presumably unwanted) cells are killed. Cytotoxic cells can be T cells, in which case the killing is antigen-specific. Natural killer (NK) cells destroy their targets in an MHC-unrestricted way. In antibody-dependent cellular cytotoxicity (ADCC), the effector cells are not HLA-specific and the antibody involved determines the specificity of the reaction.

Cytotoxic T cells (CTLs) are generally CD8$^+$ cells. They engage the target using their TcR, and the target molecules must be presented in the context of MHC class I, or in the case of alloreactivity, can be class I itself. CTLs are important in ridding the body of viruses, although a somewhat unfortunate consequence of this mechanism is that the cell harboring the virus is also removed. CTLs directed against foreign MHC class I antigens also provide a major mechanism for attacking allografts.

Natural killer activity describes the lysis of target cells in a non-MHC-restricted manner. The NK system does not appear to require priming and does not show memory. NK cells have the ability to recognize tumor cells and not normal cells and so have been implicated in cancer immunology. Natural killer cells are neither T nor B cells. From the standpoint of conventional lymphocytes, therefore, they are considered as "null" cells. However, there are some cell surface markers [such as CD16, CD56, and CD57 (NKH-1)], which are strongly associated with cells that have NK activity. Morphologically, NK cells are "large granular leukocytes" (LGLs) . The precise definition of an NK cell is open to discussion. Some believe that NK activity can be carried out by cells of different phenotypes so that the operational nature of the term NK can be preserved.

ADCC is a mechanism whereby antibody is used as a means of directing the killing of a target cell. Antibodies to cell surfaces molecules can attach to the cell by the Fab end. If the antibody is an IgG or IgM, and an NK (or K) cell is present, that cell can attach to the Fc end of the antibody molecule by means of its Fc receptors. Then the K cell causes lysis of the target. In this manner, the antibody behaves as a bridge between the target cell and the K cell, and the antibody (not the cell) dictates the specificity of the reaction. K cells, like NK cells, are also "null" and also have the appearance of LGLs. ADCC can also be mediated by eosinophils, primarily in parasitic disease. In this case, the immunoglobulin classes concerned are IgA and IgE.

B Cell Processes

B cells are less complex in their functions than T cells in that they have only one primary purpose which is to make antibodies. In addition, B cells are less fastidious in the way in which they "see" antigen. While T cells in general recognize processed antigenic peptides presented together with MHC class I or class II molecules, B cells can bind free antigen. And, if the correct set of cytokine costimulators are present, this free antigen can lead to B cell activation. In fact, many antigens are presented to B cells via APCs, but it seems that the APC may not need to process the antigen for B cells in the same ways that antigen is processed for T cells. B cell activation, like T cell activation, is a complex process involving transmembrane signaling and changes in cell morphology, phenotype, and the isotype of the antibody produced. [23] Unlike T cells, the gene rearrangements leading to the formation of complete genes for the heavy and light chains can undergo somatic mutation during the course of the antibody response. B cells use as their antigen-specific receptor the surface Ig molecules that constitute the specificity of their particular clone. (B cells can also be activated nonspecifically via mitogens. These include pokeweed mitogen (PWM) and anti- immunoglobulins. The latter stimulate B cells by crosslinking surface Ig in much the same way that anti-CD3 stimulates T cells.) Some B cells can interact directly with certain antigens, and there is apparently little if any need for APCs or auxiliary T cell activity. This is called T-independent antibody formation. It is characteristic of large antigens with repeating antigenic determinants, such as dextran. The antibody produced is mainly IgM and there is little memory. Most antigens are proteins, however. In these cases, APC activity is required, and the antigen must also activate T cells. These T cells are usually CD4$^+$, and in this capacity are called "T helper cells." The help they provide is in the form of interleukins.

Immunologic Tolerance and Suppression

Immunoregulation includes the concepts of specific as well as nonspecific modulation of immune responses, and such modulation may be stimulatory or inhibitory. Tolerance and suppression can be considered forms of inhibition or down-regulation. Immunologic tolerance is a term that denotes the failure to make a response to an immunologic stimulus. There are several aspects to consider. We are considered to be innately tolerant to self-antigens, i.e., antigens that might well evoke a response in another person (e.g., after allografting). This tolerance could exist because we do not have immunological machinery (T and/ or B cells) that react with self antigens, or because such cells, if they exist, are prevented from reacting with self antigens. Autoimmunity can be considered to be a loss of this self-tolerance, whatever the mechanism. Some experimental animals are genetic "nonresponders" to certain antigens and this too can be considered as a form of tolerance. A particularly relevant form of unresponsiveness is specific acquired immunological tolerance (SAIT). In this situation, exposure to an ordinarily immunogenic antigen (in nonimmunogenic form) leads to a state where subsequent exposure to that antigen in immunogenic form provokes little or no response. SAIT is immunologically specific.

Burnet postulated that self tolerance was established during development. A brilliant application of this principle was the experiment in 1953 where Billingham, Brent, and Medawar showed that perinatal exposure of a mouse to donor alloantigens induced a state of specific unresponsiveness so that later in life, skin allografts from the donor strain would be accepted indefinitely. [24] Thus, although later exposure to transplantation antigens leads to sensitization and rejection, very early exposure leads to tolerance. This experiment has also been done with conventional nonliving antigens.

Since that time, many facets of tolerance have emerged. As with intact animals, immature cells are easier to tolerate than mature cells. In particular, although splenic dendritic cells can activate mature thymus cells, they inactive immature thymus cells. [25] This dependence of activation on the state of maturation of a cell was postulated by Burnet to account for the loss of anti-self reactivity during development. It points out the complexity of the relation between APC and target lymphocyte in terms of eventual outcome. Antigen presentation in the periphery is also a critical factor. Thus the pathway by which antigen reaches the immunocompetent cell determines cellular processes. Some routes of antigen administration, e.g., the oral route, favor tolerance induction, whereas immunologic adjuvants make tolerance almost impossible.

The facts of these and other experiments are quite clear, but much of the basic understanding is elusive. It is clear that both T cells and B cell populations can become tolerant. T cell tolerance to many self antigens occurs by negative selection of self-reactive clones in the developing thymus. The same may be true of some developing B cells in the bone marrow.[26] However, more mature T and B cells may become unresponsive in the lymphoid periphery, a term known as *clonal anergy,* i.e., the cells are still present but do not respond to their appropriate antigens. The mechanism for inducing clonal anergy is not clear. It may occur after the presentation of excess antigen without costimulating cytokines, resulting in a "negative signal" to the cell. The clonally anergic cell would then be unresponsive to the appropriate antigen, even if it was presented in an immunogenic way.

The existence of active downregulation mechanisms became apparent when antibody modulation of the immune response was studied (see section on enhancement below). However, the existence of cell-mediated antigen-specific immunological suppression was first clearly shown in 1970 by Gershon, and it was found to be carried out by T cells. By analogy with T helpers, these have been called T suppressors (Ts), and generally carry the CD8+ phenotype. Nobody doubts the fact that all immunological processes are regulated and that there are loops of negative feedback that can be both antigen-specific and antigen-nonspecific, but the exact mechanism(s) through which the antigen-specific T cell-mediated downregulation occurs is not clear. Separate genes and gene products for antigen-specific suppressor cells have not been identified. Suppressor T cell-mediated phenomena are clearly different from more global and nonspecific immunosuppressive effects produced by cytotoxic drugs and corticosteroids. This area of research is difficult but is critical to an understanding of immunoregulation and autoimmunity.

Immunological Enhancement

This term was applied to the enhanced survival of allografts after immunological manipulation. It was first systematically investigated in animal tumor models where attempts to "vaccinate" the recipient against the tumor tissue paradoxically led to more rapid tumor growth. Enhancement can be active, in which case antigen itself is used, or it can be passive, in which case antibody is generally used.[27] Perhaps the most impressive results were generated by Stuart et al.., who were able to achieve long-term acceptance of renal allografts in rats using enhancing anti-serum.[28] However, the mechanism(s) of enhancement remain obscure and it is currently an unpopular area of research. It is mentioned at this point because of some current concepts of pregnancy immunity in which an immune response may actually enhance the survival of the fetal allograft.

Immunologic Systems

Antibody Production

Antibody production is the result of a coordinated response ultimately causing B cell activation and production of immunoglobulins. As pointed out, certain large antigens with repeating epitopes, often polysaccharides, direct a simpler form of B cell activation. In this context, APCs present antigens to the appropriate B cell clones and an IgM response occurs. The process is independent of T cells, shows little immunologic memory, and the amount of antibody is usually modest. Most antigens, however, are complex proteins. They require more sophisticated antigen-processing, and the activation of T helper cells. These, in turn, elaborate a number of cytokines that influence the magnitude and isotype of the B cell response. For instance, T cells activated by antigen produce IL-2, which in turn produces more T cell activation as well as B cell activity.

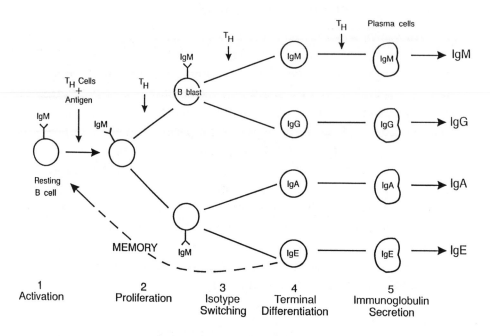

Fig. 10. B cell maturation and isotype switching is controlled at all stages by T cell signals.

The balance between the various T cell cytokines influences the isotype composition of the antibody produced. IL-4 is needed for IgE and IgG production, whereas IL-5 production favors IgA production. A schematic rendering of this process is shown in Fig. 10.

Primary antigen exposure produces a response with relatively more IgM than IgG or IgA, yet leaves the immune system "primed" in terms of having more antigen-specific T and B cells, and B cells able to make antibody of higher avidity for the antigen. Subsequent "booster" antigenic exposures thus lead to anamnestic antibody responses, which are faster in developing, larger, and of greater efficiency in combining with antigen. There are some controls over this process; repeated antigenic exposure does not necessarily lead to ever larger responses. There seems to be some "cap" on the system, although whether the negative feedback be antibody itself, anti-idiotypes, or T suppressor cell function is not clear.

Cell-Mediated Immunity (CMI): Delayed Type Hypersensitivity (DTH)

CMI is a term, often used as a synonym for DTH, which denotes a group of reactions in which T cells are the dominant cells and B cells and antibody play little or no role. Prototype examples of these reactions are the tuberculin reaction and related resistance to intracellular microorganisms, contact allergy, allograft rejection, and elimination of virally-infected cells. The antigen, presented to the cognate T cell clone, activates the T cell. This activated T cell may act in several ways. It may act directly via cell contact on an antigen-bearing target. This occurs in the case of cytolytic T cells recognizing foreign MHC or virally-infected self cells, in which the T cell receptor engages the nominal antigen in the context of class I self MHC. The target cell may be damaged via the T cell's production of cytotoxic material (called perforin or cytolysin). Or the CTL may function by inducing apoptosis (programmed cell death) in the target cell, in which case the target cell DNA fragments and the cell self-destructs.

CMI reactions can occur via the production of cytokines by the activated T cell. These can include TNF and lymphotoxin, which can damage neighbor's tissue. T cells can produce IL-2 and IFN-γ, which are capable of activating other cells, such as macrophages and NK cells to perform their functions, including destruction of intracellular microorganisms, inflammation, or killing of tumor cells.

Relations Between Cell-Mediated and Humoral Responses

It is important to recognize that although T cells can mediate CMI-DTH reactions by themselves, the immunological machinery is complex and interactive. Therefore, it is not surprising that, in vivo, complex events occur that involve both the

CMI-DTH (cellular) systems and the antibody (humoral) systems. For instance, both allograft immunity and antimicrobial immunity include CMI–DTH reactions and the production of specific antibody. Both of these reactions require APCs and specific T cells, but it is readily apparent that the activation of CD8+ T cells will trigger cytolytic processes and the activation of T helper cells of any phenotype will lead to antibody production. In the case of complex foreign tissue reactions and antimicrobial immunity, it does not follow that the epitopes recognized by the CMI–DTH system are the same to which antibody is produced. However, in the overall reaction seen in vivo, these distinctions may be difficult to recognize.

Relations
Between Humoral and Cellular Immunity

Is there any relation between the CMI-DTH reaction and antibody production in a given immunological response? Offhand, one might suspect that stronger responses would trigger both stronger CMI–DTH reactions as well as more antibody. There have been, however, provocative animal experiments showing a reciprocal relationship between CMI–DTH and antibody formation.[29] We do not know whether such regulatory interactions occur commonly in humans, but there is one outstanding example in leprosy. It is clear that there is an inverse relation between the strength of the lepromatous reactions and the tuberculoid reactions in human disease.[30] Patients with tuberculoid lesions have high levels of DTH to leprosy antigens, few mycobacteria in the lesions, and little or no antimycobacterial antibodies. In contrast, lepromatous lesions are swarming with mycobacteria and there is antibody but not DTH to mycobacterial antigens.

The underlying basis for these reciprocal relations between humoral and cell-mediated immunity probably lies in the types of T cell subsets and their cytokines that are involved in the two discordant processes.[22]

Allograft Reactions

Historically, classical immunology described allograft reactions that were antigen specific and directed to MHC specificities. In skin grafting systems across the MHC, the initial graft is rejected in "first set" fashion, meaning a moderately paced inflammatory reaction that occurs over a period of 10–20 days. However, the systemic result of such a process is the specific sensitization of the recipient so that a second graft bearing the same MHC antigens is rejected in a "second set" or accelerated fashion, e.g., over 7–12 days. This is an example of "positive immunologic memory" and is analogous, in the T cell system, to the anamnestic response in antibody-mediated reactions. The immunologic memory is antigen-specific, because a second graft containing different MHC antigens will be rejected in first-set fashion.

The allograft reactions are primarily mounted by CD4$^+$ and CD8$^+$ T cells, which recognize and respond to class II and class I MHC antigens, respectively, on the foreign graft. They may act directly on grafted cells as CTL or trigger DTH reactions by stimulating inflammatory cells. However, there is an antibody response that also occurs in responses to allografts. It may not be readily apparent in first- and second-set reactions, but continued exposure to the same MHC can raise sufficient antibody so that a graft is immediately rejected before vascularization takes place, via antibody and complement damage to the endothelium. This results in a "white graft reaction" seen in skin transplants and in the hyperacute rejection occasionally seen in kidney, liver, and heart transplants.[31]

Mucosal Immune Systems

When it was discovered that instead of IgG, a special form of IgA, secretory IgA, was the predominant immunoglobulin isotype in gastrointestinal secretions, it became evident that the mammalian immune system was not uniformly constructed. Instead, there were anatomical and physiologic subdivisions with distinct characteristics. These features include specialized expression of immunoglobulin isotypes, of T cell receptors, of lymphoid migratory patterns, and of mast cell subsets.[32] These distinctive mechanisms are added to the nonspecific protective materials present at mucosal interfaces, such as mucous secretion, ciliary clearance, low gastric pH, lysozyme, and so on. Because of these peculiarities, not represented within the "classical" immunological machinery, as typified by the spleen and deep lymph nodes, several loosely defined mucosal immune systems have been identified. These are the gut-associated lymphoid system (GALT) and the bronchus-associated lymphoid system (BALT). One might consider the mucosal immune system of the genitourinary tract as well, although much less work has been done on this system than on the GALT and BALT systems.

One of the salient features of the gut and bronchus-associated lymphoid systems is that they are constantly being confronted with an extraordinary panoply of environmental antigens coming to them via ingestion and respiration. (This constant exposure to environmental antigens is a property of the skin as well, and some investigators have also distinguished the skin-associated lymphoid system [SALT] as another "mucosal type" subdivision of the immune system.) Pathways have developed to cope with this antigenic onslaught, but only a few features can be described here.

Secretory IgA differs from the predominant form of circulating IgA. The latter is composed of two a heavy chains and two light chains. Secretory IgA is a dimer consisting of two pairs of the heavy-light chain units plus a J chain and a secretory piece. The latter two additions make secretory IgA resistant to proteolytic digestion that would otherwise occur in the gut. The switch to the IgA isotype is regulated by T cells via IL-5 and other cytokines, but the location of IgA producing B cells is specially arranged. B cell precursors are enriched in Peyer's patches in the intestine. After meeting antigen, they move to regional lymph nodes and then back to the more diffuse mucosal lymphoid tissue. As they complete this circuit, they terminally differentiate into plasma cells secreting IgA.

Other characteristics of mucosal lymphoid tissue is a relative increase of T cells bearing αδ receptors and a preponderance of mast cells that contain chondroitin sulfate-E rather than heparin. The precise significance of these characteristics is as yet unknown.

The immunological response of the female genital tract to antigens is pertinent to the focus of this book. It is understandable that most of the available data have been gathered through animal studies and that, because of the importance of humoral defenses in microbial infection, the emphasis has been on antibody formation rather than on cell-mediated immunity. The subject is additionally complex because the response of various parts of the genital tract (vagina, cervix, uterus) may differ, and sex hormones have a significant impact on local humoral immunity.

Immunoglobulin concentrations in genital secretions are intermediate between those in plasma and those in the gut. There is IgG and monomeric IgA as well as secretory IgA. Hormonal changes influence the immune variables. Cervical mucus IgG and IgA are highest at the preovulatory phase and in the luteal phase and lowest at the time of the LH peak.[33] Antibody responses can be induced in the genital tract by direct intravaginal antigen presentation. Systemic immunization can also result in genital antibodies either because of serum transudation or because of B lymphocyte migration to the mucosal surfaces. The cellular component of the genital immune system will be discussed in Chapter 4.

Summary

1. The immune system is designed to discriminate between self and nonself, and to mount defensive processes against nonself.
2. The immune system is characterized by *specificity, memory, mobility, replicability, and cooperativity.*
3. It operates via antigen-specific and antigen-nonspecific pathways.

4. The antigen-specific paths include T cells and B cells and B cell products, i.e., immunoglobulins. Immunoglobulin antibodies may be anti-antigen or anti-antibody (anti-idiotype).

   a. T cells and B cells, with their antigen-specific receptors, are clonally selected via a series of gene rearrangements, mutations, and selection.

   b. T cells and B cells have a series of surface markers that are important in their function and that can also serve to distinguish them and their states of differentiation.

5. Nonspecific aspects of the immune response include macrophages and other antigen-presenting cells, inflammatory cells, and the complement system.

6. Both specific and nonspecific pathways communicate both by direct cellular interactions and by means of *cytokines*.

7. The major histocompatibility complex (MHC) products are critical both for self-recognition and alloreactivity.

8. Cellular processes in the immune response include:

   a. Antigen presentation;

   b. Cellular activation, proliferation, and differentiation;

   c. Cytotoxicity; and

   d. Immunoglobulin production.

9. Immunologic suppression or downregulation is critical in controlling immune processes. Although poorly understood, it can involve specific T cells and nonspecific pathways as well.

10. The final effects of activation of the immune system include:

    a. Antibody production both local and systemic, of a variety of isotypes;

    b. Cell-mediated immunity and delayed hypersensitivity;

    c. Allograft rejection.

11. The programming of the immune system's processes are controlled and integrated.

References

1. Abbas A-K, Lichtman AH, Pober JS: *Cellular and Molecular Immunology*, Philadelphia, W.B. Saunders; 1991.
2. Klein J: *Immunology*, Boston, Blackwell Scientific; 1990.
3. Paul WE: *Fundamental Immunology*, New York, Raven Press; 1989.
4. Strober W, Brown WR: The mucosal immune system, in Samter M, Talmage DW, Frank MM, Austen KF, Claman HN (eds): *Immunological Diseases*, Fourth edition. Boston, Little, Brown and Company; 1988.
5. Roitt IM: *Essential Immunology*, Oxford, Blackwell Scientific; 1988.
6. Stites DP, Terr AI: *Basic and Clinical Immunology*, Norwalk, CT, Appleton & Lange; 1991.
7. Ashwell JD, Klausner RD: Genetic and mutational analysis of the T-cell antigen receptor. *Annu Rev Immunol* 1990; 8:139–167.
8. Marrack P, Kappler JW: The antigen-specific, major histo-compatibility complex-restricted receptor on T cells. *Adv Immunol* 1986; 38: 1–30.
9. Williams AF, Barclay AN: The immunoglobulin superfamily - domains for cell surface recognition. *Ann Rev Immunol* 1988; 6: 381–405.
10. Raulet DH: The structure, function and molecular genetics of the γ/δ T cell receptor. *Ann Rev Immunol* 1989; 7: 175–208.
11. diGiovine FS, Duff GW: Interleukin-1: The first interleukin. *Immunol Today* 1990; 11: 13–20.
12. Arai K, Lee F, Miyajima, et al.: Cytokines: Coordinators of immune and inflammatory responses. *Annu Rev Biochem* 1990; 59: 783–836.
13. Nicola NA: Hematopoietic cell growth factors and their receptors. *Annu Rev Biochem* 1989; 58: 45–77.
14. French DL, Laskov R, Scharff MD: The role of somatic hypermutation in the generation of antibody diversity. *Science* 1989; 244: 1152–1157.
15. Alt FW, Blackwell TK, Yancopoulos GD: Development of the primary antibody repertoire. *Science* 1987; 238: 1079–1087.

16. Kohler H, Urbain J, Casenave PA: *Idiotypy in Biology and Medicine*, New York, Academic Press; 1984.
17. Hunkapiller T, Hood L: Diversity of the immunoglobulin gene superfamily. *Adv Immunol* 1989; 44: 1–63.
18. Harding CV, Unanue ER: Cellular mechanisms of antigen processing and the function of class I and class II major histocompatibility complex molecules. *Cell Regul* 1990; 1: 499–509.
19. Monaco JJ: A molecular model of MHC class-I-restricted antigen processing. *Immunol Today* 1992; 13: 173–178.
20. Marrack P, Kappler JW: The staphylococcal enterotoxins and their relatives. *Science* 1990; 248: 705–712.
21. Weksler ME, Moody CE, Kozak RW: The autologous mixed-lymphocyte reaction. *Adv Immunol* 1981; 31: 271–312.
22. Bloom BR, Modlin RL, Salgame P: Stigma variations: Observations on suppressor T cells and leprosy. *Ann Rev Immunol* 1992; 10: 453–488.
23. Clark EA, Lane PJL: Regulation of human B-cell activation and adhesion. *Ann Rev Immunol* 1991; 9: 97–127.
24. Billingham RE, Brent L, Medawar PB: "Actively acquired tolerance" of foreign cells. *Nature* 1953; 172: 603–606.
25. Matzinger P, Guerder S: Does T-cell tolerance require a dedicated antigen-presenting cell? *Nature* 1989; 338: 74–76.
26. Nemazee DA, Burki K: Clonal deletion of B lymphocytes in a transgeneic mouse bearing anti-MHC class I antibody genes. *Nature* 1989; 337: 562–566.
27. Voisin GA: Role of antibody classes in the regulatory facilitation reaction. *Immunol Rev* 1980; 49: 3–59.
28. Stuart FP, McKearn TJ, Weiss A, et al.: Suppression of rat renal allograft rejection by antigen and antibody. *Immunol Rev* 1980; 49: 127–165.
29. Parish CR: The relationship between humoral and cell-mediated immunity. *Transplant Rev* 1972; 13: 35–63.
30. Hastings RC: *Leprosy*, Edinburgh, Churchill-Livingstone; 1985.
31. Mason DW, Morris PJ: Effector mechanisms in allograft rejection. *Ann Rev Immunol* 1986; 4: 119–145.

32. Strober W, Brown WR: The mucosal immune system, in Samter M, Talmage DW, Frank MM, Austen KF, Claman HN (eds): *Immunological Diseases,* Fourth edition. Boston, Little, Brown & Co.; 1988: 79–139.

33. Schumacher GFB: Humoral immune factors in the female reproductive tract and their changes during the cycle, in Dhindsa DS, Schumacher GFB (eds): *Immunological Aspects of Infertility and Fertility Regulation.* NY, Elsevier/North Holland; 1980: 93–141.

Chapter 2

Materno–Fetal Relationships

Immunological Aspects

Components of the Materno–Fetal Interface

The subjects of interest in this chapter are the immunological aspects of the interface between maternal tissue in the decidua and allogeneic fetal tissue in the trophoblast. It is obvious, however, that as pregnancy proceeds, the two tissues become so intimately intermingled that identification of a particular cell as originally being fetal or maternal can be impossible.

A detailed description of the development of the embryo from the fertilized ovum is not required for an analysis of this topic. Nonetheless, an understanding of certain aspects of placental structure is crucial for interpreting the immunological aspects of pregnancy.

Structure of the Trophoblast

It is useful to distinguish between the villous trophoblast and the nonvillous trophoblast, both of which are derived from the fetus. A principal point of contact between the fetal and maternal tissues exists in or near the chorionic villi. These projections of fetal tissue are covered by two layers. The outer layer (facing the maternal component) is the *syncytiotrophoblast* —a nonmitotic covering that once consisted of individual cells

but that has matured into an acellular syncytium.[1] This layer
also lines the intervillous blood spaces. Beneath the syncytiotrophoblast is the *cytotrophoblast,* also called the Langhans cell
layer. This layer is more metabolically active than the
syncytiotrophoblast. Some cytotrophoblast cells push through
the syncytiotrophoblast to make *cytotrophoblast columns* that
help to join the villi to the maternal tissue. Some cytotrophoblast
cells break away from the columns to form the *cytotrophoblast
shell,* and some of these cells migrate into the myometrium where
they are called *interstitial cytotrophoblast* cells. Furthermore,
some cytotrophoblast cells invade the spiral arteries of the uterus
and line the vessels as *endovascular trophoblast.*[2] (These cells
are probably the source of the cells that break off and embolize
the maternal systemic circulation, a phenomenon known as
trophoblast deportation [Chapter 4].)

The nonvillous trophoblast comprises the rest of the
trophoblastic tissue. From it develop other parts of the placenta,
including the chorion laeve and chorionic plate, the marginal
zone, and the basal plate. Benirschke points out that there is
confusion in the nomenclature, and prefers the term *extravillous
trophoblast* to nonvillous trophoblast.[1]

HLA Expression on the Trophoblast

Whether the materno–fetal interface contains parental transplantation antigens and whether there is any maternal recognition of
such antigens (if present) are central matters in interpreting the immunological paradox of pregnancy. If the trophoblast does not exhibit paternal HLA antigens (with or without maternal HLA antigens)
then indeed there is a "no-man's land," immunologically speaking,
and maternal T cells are not directly confronted with allogeneic
tissue. If, however, there are paternal HLA antigens on the trophoblast, then one must explain how it is that maternal T cell activity
directed toward paternal antigens does not develop, at least not in
sufficient quantity to abort the fetus.

Experiments have been done that support both sides of the argument. Some workers had results that indicated that HLA is present; others did not show HLA on the trophoblast. The "real" answer, which includes an explanation for the experimental discrepancies, was a surprise to both sides of the controversy. It should also be pointed out that although the correct answer to this classic problem had been suspected for some time, it required newer techniques such as the development of monoclonal antibodies and molecular biological techniques to prove it.

In a classic investigation in 1962, Simmons and Russell studied the antigenicity of the trophoblast in mice.[3] They transplanted trophoblast tissue and embryos (without trophoblast) into allogeneic hosts. The trophoblasts survived even in a presensitized host, but the embryos did not. Therefore they believed that the trophoblast was weak or lacking in antigenicity. This belief is indeed strengthened by the failure of rejection of the trophoblast in the sensitized environment, because work to be reviewed in the next chapter on the question of the immunologically privileged status of the uterus, shows that MHC-containing tissues are almost always rejected by sensitized hosts, even if placed in "privileged sites." Simmons and Russell concluded from their important functional studies that histocompatibility antigens (about which little was known in 1962) were either absent from the trophoblast or were not expressed in an immunogenic manner.

When reagents became available that could identify human MHC antigens by immunohistochemical means, these reagents were used to explore MHC expression in the placenta. Faulk and Temple[4] showed that antibodies to β_2 microglobulin and to HLA-A2 stained the cells within the chorionic villi but did not stain the surface layers of the trophoblast. Since both of these antigens are markers for HLA class I histocompatibility antigens, this may be the first study showing that these components of the MHC are selectively absent from the villous trophoblast. Later, other workers showed that HLA class II (DR) antigens could be found within the stroma of the placenta but not on the trophoblast.[5]

When the components of the extravillous trophoblast were similarly studied, the results were somewhat different. Extravillous trophoblast stained strongly with anti-HLA class I antibodies, such as W6/32, yet they failed to stain with antibodies to antigens specific for paternal antigens.[6,7] This puzzling discrepancy was resolved by the recognition that the antibodies that did stain trophoblast cells were antibodies against the nonpolymorphic (invariant) parts of the HLA molecule. By contrast, the antibodies that did not stain trophoblast cells were directed against the individual HLA specificities expressed on the amino-terminal ends of the molecules.

These findings raised the possibility that the HLA molecules found on extravillous trophoblast may be unusual in some way. Several possibilities were mentioned. They might be "masked" by some covering material so that they would not be accessible either to the maternal T cells or to anti-HLA reagents used for identification. They might be in some peculiar physical configuration so that their immunogenicity was altered or lost. They might turn out to be members of a primitive HLA family that had not developed genetic polymorphisms,[7] although it has been those very polymorphisms that have made MHC genes and gene products of such extraordinary interest. This latter possibility has some intriguing implications. If there are MHC-type molecules on the trophoblast that are not polymorphic, they will not be recognized as foreign by the maternal T cell system.

In 1986–1987, it was discovered that the region of the sixth chromosome that contained the MHC class I genes had more genes than those responsible for the known HLA A, B, and C products. Although this multigene family contained some pseudogenes (i.e., genes that are not transcribed) it also encoded three previously unrecognized gene products, now called HLA E, F, and G.[8] Basically, these are genes with very high homologies with classical HLA class I genes but that are truncated.[9,10] The gene products do associate with B_2 microglobulin and so comprise a somewhat different kind of HLA class I molecule. HLA-G α

Table 1
Antigens Present on Human Trophoblast Cells

	Extravillous Cytotrophoblast	Villous Cytotrophoblast	Syncytiotrophoblast
MHC molecules			
Class I			
HLA-A,B	—a	—a	—
HLA-G	yes[a]	yes±	—
Class II			
HLA-DR	—	—	—
Complement regulatory molecules			
Membrane cofactor protein (MCP) CD46	yes	yes	yes
Receptors			
Fcγ receptor	?	?	yes
IL-2 receptor	—	—	—

[a]Extravillous and villous cytotrophoblast contains class I (HLA-A,B) mRNA and HLA-G mRNA *(15)*.

chains are prominent in the cytotrophoblasts in the first and second trimester. They are also present in some (but not all) choriocarcinomas.[11] The important point is that these HLA molecules, of which HLA G is the best studied, show very little, if any, polymorphism.[10] Since HLA-G is not found on normal lymphoid cells, it is not related to the concept of TLX antigens *(see below).* Thus most, if not all, of the HLA molecules expressed on the trophoblast are HLA G. The current state of knowledge is shown in Table 1. The HLA-G molecules are present early in pregnancy and their levels decline as pregnancy advances.

Regulation of HLA Expression

The presence and/or amount of HLA expression on a cell reflects a variety of processes, not all of which are well understood. Although it is commonly stated that all diploid, nucleated human cells express MHC molecules codominantly, this is not universally true. A number of tissues lack class I HLA, including cerebral cortex and cerebellum, sympathetic ganglia, pituitary, thyroid and parathyroid cells, and hepatocytes.[12] There are interesting data on this point with regard to germ cells and early preimplantation embryos. The question of whether mature spermatozoa carry MHC antigens has yielded very conflicting opinions.[13] The consensus opinion is that few if any HLA molecules are integral to the surface of sperm cells, yet the possibility exists that some HLA antigens from the semen may be adsorbed onto spermatozoa. (Whether such "adoptively acquired" HLA specificities have practical significance is as yet unknown.) In similar experiments on human oocytes and zona pellucida, immunohistochemical staining failed to show the presence of HLA class I or class II molecules.[13]

Exactly when MHC molecules become expressed by the fetus or the trophoblast is not known. Preimplantation embryos do not stain for HLA antigens,[14] but MHC antigens have been seen in the yolk sac as early as 3 weeks of gestation.[13] We do not know at which point between the 8-cell stage and the 3-week stage HLA expression becomes evident.

The regulation of MHC gene expression involves complicated processes.[12] When the genes are present, expression of the gene product can be controlled via the production of mRNA (transcriptional control), or via the production of protein (translational control). Control mechanisms are important in HLA-G gene activation. The HLA-G gene is transcribed in normal villous and extravillous trophoblast, but not in syncytiotrophoblast.[15] The villous trophoblast can translate the transcribed message into expressed protein.[9] Recent work using *in situ* hybridization has shown that HLA-G mRNA can be detected in first trimester cytotrophoblast and in term chorionic membrane cytotrophoblast. In contrast, HLA-G mRNA was only seen in very low amounts or was undetectable in syncytiotrophoblast cells, whether from first or third trimester placentas.[16] Thus, transcription of the HLA-G gene is seen in the cytotrophoblast but not in the syncytiotrophoblast.

The expression of HLA gene products on the cell surface may vary. It appears not to change in various phases of the cell cycle, but it can be upregulated. Cytokines, specifically interferons, can increase HLA class I expression. This can be shown either by adding interferons to cell cultures or by inducing interferon production through virus infection.[12] Class II MHC molecules are also upregulated via IFN-γ exposure.[17] In terms of allorecognition in pregnancy, can interferons or similar substances, perhaps induced by inflammation, upregulate HLA expression? This might occur in low-HLA expressing cells. It is even possible that cells that express no HLA might be persuaded to do so under the right circumstances. However, it is extremely interesting that the trophoblast may be different from other peripheral tissues because there are reports that IFN-γ does not increase the expression of HLA-A, -B, -C, or -G in villous trophoblast.[15,18,19] This could be an extremely important fail-safe mechanism in materno–fetal allorecognition, tending to diminish the effectiveness of any alloreactive cells that might be poised to interact destructively with MHC-bearing trophoblast cells.

Other Antigens Present at the Materno–Fetal Interface

A variety of antigens and antigenic systems have been identified in the placenta. Some of these are interesting from the standpoint of the immunology of pregnancy and some are not. Those of interest would naturally include polymorphic systems (other than MHC) because their existence would allow the possibility of allogeneic differences between mother and fetus, and the consequence of such allogeneic encounters might be important for the success or failure of pregnancy itself. Examples

of such nonMHC polymorphic systems are the erythrocyte antigenic systems (ABO, P, Rh, and others), placental alkaline phosphatase and possibly the trophoblast–leukocyte crossreacting
(TLX) system. Some placental antigens may not indeed function
as antigens in the above sense, i.e., by invoking an immune
response, but are called antigens because they are identified by
marker antibodies and are important in the functioning of the
immune response. Such molecules include receptors for the Fc
segments of immunoglobulins (FcRs) and targets for immun-
logically competent elements such as natural killer (NK) cells.
The cellular smorgasbord of immunoreactant cells themselves
will be covered in the next subsection.

TLX antigens and antibodies. There has been a great deal
of interest in whether there are polymorphic antigenic systems,
independent of HLA, that might influence the course or outcome
of human pregnancy. A candidate system is the *trophoblast–
leukocyte cross reacting* (TLX) system of Faulk and colleagues.[20]
These investigators raised a series of rabbit antisera against human
trophoblast tissue. Such antibodies reacted with trophoblast but
also with decidual stroma and the endothelium of chorionic villi
as well as with peripheral blood leukocytes (PBL), and some
human cell lines. When the antisera were adsorbed with PBL,
they no longer reacted with PBL, stroma, or villous endothelium
but still reacted with trophoblast and some cell lines. Thus, the
original interpretation was that the antisera contained a mixture
of antibodies (which was reasonable, as they were xenoantisera).
The investigators proposed the existence of two trophoblastic
antigenic (TA) systems; TA-1 antigens, which are present on
the trophoblast and certain cell lines, and TA-2 antigens, which
are present on PBL and placental endothelium. The investigators
were particularly intrigued by the possibility that the TLX system
and the HLA system were involved in the different outcomes
seen in normal pregnancy vs recurrent spontaneous abortion
(RSAb). The argument that was then developed was heavily
influenced by the idea (then prevalent) that HLA sharing between

father and mother was a very significant variable, often leading
to RSAb. (The concept that HLA sharing is important in RSAb
has been reevaluated; Chapter 6.)

The hypothesis stated that because the TLX system might
be polymorphic, normal pregnancy led to the development of
maternal antifetal TLX antibodies of the TA-2 variety. If there
was also little or no HLA sharing, then pregnancy advanced. If
there was excess HLA sharing, than the protective effect of the
allogeneic difference "failed," and TA-2 antibodies were not
produced but instead TA-1 antibodies were made. These
antibodies, directed against the trophoblast antigens, caused the
pregnancy to abort. Thus, TA-2 antibodies functioned as
significant *blocking antibodies,* inhibiting recognition of, or
cytotoxicity to TA-1 antigens.[20] Therefore, RSAb was associated
with *the absence of a protective blocking factor,* i.e., anti-TA-2.
This concept was reminiscent of the work of Rocklin and
colleagues who had recently noted the absence of a serum factor
in women with RSAb. This factor was believed to block maternal
antifetal reactions and was present in normal pregnancy.[21]

A number of papers about the TLX system have been put
forth by Faulk and McIntyre and colleagues, and the results and
interpretations have been widely quoted. When the 10 TLX
antibodies were tested against PBL from a random panel of 30
HLS-typed donors, some TLX antibodies recognized some PBL,
whereas other antibodies recognized different PBL. There was
considerable overlap, and there was no correlation between the
pattern of recognition by the different TLX antibodies and the
HLA types of the PBL target cells.[22] Therefore, anti-TLX
antibodies are not anti-HLA, nor do they seem to be linked to
observable HLA antigens. The differing patterns of reactivity of
the 10 antisera led to the belief that the TLX system was
polymorphic. A subsequent publication covered much of the
same material. At this point, the investigators believed that there
were three groups of TLX antigens. Groups 1 and 3 were
independent, whereas group 2 was a combination of 1 and 3.[23]

By 1986, a monoclonal antibody, H316, had been obtained that recognized structures on human trophoblasts, PBL, and some tumor cells, including choriocarcinoma and teratocarcinoma.[24] Thus it was possibly directed to TLX antigens. Exactly what antigens were being bound by H316 was not known, but data were developed to show that the antibody bound glycoproteins of 55 and 65 kDa mol wt. However, H316 was not alloreactive, and it did not block MLRs. These results agree with the concept that anti-TLX are not anti-MHC, but if MLRs are not blocked, then one can ask what the relevance of this anti-TLX antibody to materno–fetal alloreactivity may be. The schema for TLX activity was subsequently revised.[25] All pregnancies generated anti-TLX antibodies.These would appear to be injurious if not blocked or neutralized. However, the anti-TLX antibodies caused the production of anti-idiotypic antibodies (anti-anti-TLX). Or, in idiotype language, antibody-1 (anti-TLX) provokes production of antibody-2 (anti-anti-TLX). How these antibodies are related to the originally described TA-1 and TA-2[20] is not clear. The antigen-antibody complexes [antibody-1 - antibody-2] somehow control maternal recognition of the fetus, and the presence of these complexes neutralizes the capacity of anti-TLX (antibody-1) to produce tissue damage. Studies with 10 new rabbit anti-TLX antisera found that there was no cytotoxicity against T cells from 10 normal donors, but all 10 antisera killed B cells, albeit at fairly high concentrations. A panel analysis seemed to show some specificity, but a larger group of PBL may be needed to prove alloreactive polymorphism of anti-TLX antibodies.[26] The investigators believed that the TLX system contained poly-morphic determinants but admitted that none of the three mouse monoclonal anti-TLX antibodies then available showed any alloreactive specificity. Perhaps they were directed to mono-morphic epitopes in the TLX system. More recently, immuno-chemical analysis of the binding of one of these monoclonal antibodies led to the identification of a 35 kDa protein from PBLs reacting with anti-TLX.[27] This result was not similar to previous work where the proteins identified by H316 were said to be 55 and 65 kDa.[28] The latest development concerns the identification of the specific targets for the monoclonal antibodies, H316 and GB24. Each of these appears to recognize a different epitope on the same molecule, and the molecule has been identified as membrane cofactor protein (MCP).[29] MCP is a member of a group of proteins that regulate activation of the complement system. It is recognized as CD46 and is present on a number of cells including trophoblast, sperm, and leukocytes. Therefore, although it is by definition a TLX antigen, there is no compelling data that it is polymorphic.

The idea that there is some important non-HLA polymorphic system of transplantation antigens is attractive in principle, and is congruent with statements that all successful pregnancies have circulating antibodies suppressing the mother's response to paternal antigens,[30] but there are unanswered questions, partucularly with the TLX system, which is the leading contender in this field. For instance, there are few confirmed reports that anti-TLX antibodies or complexes containing these antibodies have been recovered from human pregnancy sera.[25] The whole subject "needs to be cleared up".[31] Table 1 shows a consensus of the location of HLA and the putative TLX antigens in the trophoblast.

The *erythrocyte blood group antigens,* particularly those of the ABO and Rh systems, are of considerable interest in the immunology of pregnancy because of the potential for isoimmunization and the development of hemolytic disease of the newborn (Chapter 5). Aside from those considerations, however, it is pertinent to the problems of differential gene activation and gene product expression to understand whether such antigens are present in the placenta. Both the A and B blood group substances are not found on the trophoblast,[32] but Rh (D) is present. This is a curious fact whose significance escapes us. However, since it is generally recognized that maternal sensitization by Rh antigens of the fetus occurs around the time of placental disruption at delivery, it is clear that the mere presence of Rh (D) alloantigens on the trophoblast existing in the uterus of an RH (D) negative mother is not sufficient to lead to anti-D production. This fact may be related to the concept that MHC class II antigens are necessary for antigen presentation to helper T cells, and thus to subsequent antibody production. Thus, the lack of MHC class II at the materno-fetal interface may account for the failure of trophoblast Rh (D) to sensitize.

A placental isoenzyme of *alkaline phosphatase (PLAP)* is found on syncytiotrophoblast but not on most other trophoblast cells.[33] There is some genetic polymorphism with regard to this enzyme, but maternal antibodies to PLAP have not been found.[34] Furthermore, as it is not seen until after the first trimester, it is not likely to be critical in immunoregulation at the materno–fetal interface. The function of PLAP is not known, but it may be related to growth regulation.

Receptors for immunoglobulins are present in the placenta. As with such proteins in general, they bind to the constant regions of immunoglobulin molecules in the Fc region, and thus are called Fc receptors (FcRs) The prominent FcR in the placenta binds to the constant region of the γ chain of IgG and is termed FcRγ. It is critical for the transplacental passage of maternal IgG.

NK target structures and other molecules may be important in pathways where MHC-specific mechanisms do not operation. NonMHC restricted cell damage must be considered in systems where graft rejection is a possibility. Mechanisms for MHC-unrestricted cell killing include natural killer (NK) and lymphokine-activated killer (LAK) pathways. The structure of the actual target of NK activity on the NK susceptible cell is not known, but functional studies can determine if such targets are present. Recent work has shown that although NK cells are present in the decidua, there does not seem to be any lysis when such cells are added to human culture trophoblast cells. The interpretation (although not the only possible one) is that the trophoblast cells do not have NK target structures on their surfaces and so are resistant to NK mediated lysis. Similar studies using human trophoblastic tumor cell lines have also shown that they are not susceptible to MHC-nonrestricted lysis by LAK cells induced by culturing PBLs in IL-2.[35]

Cellular Constituents of Placental Tissue

One can approach the immunological aspects of the materno–fetal interface in yet another way, i.e., by describing the types of non-trophoblast cells in the placenta and the kinds of surface molecules on those cells. This method of phenotypic analysis has been made easier by the development of monoclonal antibodies that can be used in immunochemical studies or in flow cytometry. Furthermore, since reagents are now available that can detect cytokines and cytokine receptors, these essentially morphological methods can provide insight into the nature of functional pathways.

Maternal cells in the placenta can be divided into several categories. These include what might be called "traditional" immunological cells, i.e., lymphocytes and macrophages, and also "nontraditional" but currently accepted immunologic cells, i.e., large granular leukocytes (LGLs). However, it should be recognized that there are special problems in the analysis of placental cell populations. For instance, there are cells that seem peculiar to placental tissue, such as Kornchenzellen (K) cells and X cells. As these cells do not seem to have exact counterparts elsewhere in the body, their characterization is difficult. In addition, the distribution patterns of surface markers on placental cells, even cells that do have counterparts elsewhere in the body (such as lymphocytes) are not always the same as those seen in those counterparts.

The decidua contains an abundance of macrophages, which are MHC class II+ and CD14[+].[36] These cells can present antigen to T cells and, as effector cells, can perform phagocytic and other functions, including the secretion of the immunosuppressive material, PGE-2.

The analysis of T cell populations in the placenta poses some problems. The majority of the mature T cells in peripheral blood and peripheral tissues are either $CD2^+$, $CD3^+$, $CD4^+$ (commonly called T helper [Th] cells), or are $CD2^+$, $CD3^+$, $CD8^+$ (commonly called T cytotoxic/suppressor [Tc/s] cells). Since the CD3 molecule is intimately connected with the T cell receptor (TcR) for antigen, these Th and Tc/s cells are clonally selected and antigen-sensitive. Decidual T cells may be different. Some studies have described cells that are $CD2^+$ but $CD3^-$, $CD4^-$, $CD8^-$.[37] This phenotype suggests that the cell is either not a T cell or it is a very primitive T cell. If it is a T cell, the absence of CD3 implies the absence of the TcR; hence, such cells would not be specifically antigen-reactive or alloreactive (although they might be activatible by other means). More conventional T cell profiles have been seen, for instance $CD3^+$, $CD4^+$, and $CD3^+$, $CD8^+$.[36] In this study, it was interesting that there were relatively more $CD8^+$ than $CD4^+$ cells. This is the inverse of what is seen in the blood and peripheral tissues and, according to the conventional wisdom, could indicate a preponderance of cytotoxic/suppressor activity over helper activity.

The cells mentioned above that have some markers characteristic of T cells, e.g., $CD2^+$, but which are $CD3^-$, $CD4^-$, and $CD8^-$ [6] arise early in pregnancy and their distribution is similar to that of K cells. K cells have been recognized for years, but the nomenclature has been confusing. K cells have been called metrial cells. Because they are full of granules they have also been called stromal granulocytes.[38] This term is rather unfortunate as it leads one, by associative thinking, to consider K cells as related to polymorphonuclear (granular) leukocytes. Perhaps it is better to call these cells uterine large granular leukocytes (U-LGL).[39] A consensus among the available data indicates that the staining profile of U-LGL cells is $CD2^+$, $CD3^-$, $CD16^-$, $CD45^+$, $CD56^+$, $CD57^+$ (HNK-1$^+$).[36,38,39] Morphologically they are large granular leukocytes. They may resemble NK cells (which are LGLs), but U-LGL cells stain for certain NK cell markers ($CD56^+$, $CD57^+$,

[HNK-1[+]]) and not for others (CD16[-]).[40] This apparent discrepancy is not bothersome for the present writer as he has always considered the term "NK" to describe an operational function and not a particular type of cell. (This means that NK activity may well be carried out by cells of different phenotypes.) U-LGL cells do have NK activity against conventional NK targets, such as the tumor line, K562[36,41] but, as we have seen, the trophoblast itself seems to resist NK mediated lysis. U-LGL mitotic activity increases from proliferative phase through late secretory phase of the menstrual cycle.[42] This indicates that U-LGL cells are not endstage cells and that their number and activities are hormonally controlled. If pregnancy does not occur, they lessen in number, whereas if pregnancy ensues, they increase.[43] Such cells may also secrete factors that suppress mitogen responses (*see* Chapter 3). One might easily postulate important antiproliferative roles for U-LGLs in the decidua.

NK cells have come under considerable scrutiny. They decrease in number and activity in the peripheral blood in pregnancy, but their function does not change in the decidua. NK activity in the decidua is less than that in peripheral blood, but can be raised to that level in vitro if IL-2 is added. (It is paradoxical that IL-2 receptors were not increased in this situation.[44]) The role of NK cells in possibly downregulating maternal antifetal reactions is not yet clear. NK cells are not essential for pregnancy in mice, as NK-deficient animals have offspring.[44] Perhaps the most interesting point is that expression of the HLA-G α chain protein in HLA-A, -B, and -C null cells reduced their susceptibility to NK and γδ T cell mediated lysis.[11]

A comparison of the cell surface markers of peripheral T and NK cells and uterine LGL's is shown in Table 2.

The study of cytokines in the placenta is just starting. In this respect, it is pertinent to look at IL-1 for its role in macrophage metabolism, at IL-2 for its activity in T cell and B cell stimulation and at IFN-γ for its ability to stimulate NK activity and MHC class II expression.

Table 2
Antigenic Profiles of T Natural Killer (NK)
and Uterine Large Granular Leukocytes (U-LGL)

	Leukocyte Surface Antigens			
	CD2	CD3	CD4	CD8
Peripheral T cells				
"Helper" T	+	+	+	
"Cytotoxic/ suppressor" T	+	+		+
Peripheral NK cells				
Decidual U-LGLs	+			
	CD16	CD45	CD56	CD57
Peripheral T cells				
"Helper" T				
"Cytotoxic/ suppressor" T				
Peripheral NK cells	+	+	+	+
Decidual U-LGLs		+	+	+

IL-1 has been demonstrated in placental tissues[45] but it may not be able to exert all of its usual panoply of effects—the data are not clear. There are suggestions that IL-2 activity may be deficient in the placenta,[45] and decidual T cells were found to be negative for CD25.[36] Since CD25 is part of the IL-2 receptor, this implies that placental T cells may not become activated and proliferate in response to IL-2 unless some means (IL-1?) is found to upregulate their IL-2 receptors. The low levels of NK activity in decidual cells (compared with PBL) can be increased in culture by adding IL-2.[40,41] CD56+ and CD56- cells proliferate when IL-2 is added, but they don't make any IL-2 themselves.[41] IL-2 added to placental mononuclear cells will increase the production of IFN-γ and increase the LAK activity and maintain the NK activity of these cells.[46] Taken together, these early data imply that some aspects of cytokine production and regulation are not the same in the placenta as they are in peripheral lymphoid tissues.

Furthermore, other cytokine systems will have to be studied. Both IL-3 and GM-CSF stimulate the proliferation of cultured placental cells, at least in the mouse.[47] Probes are now available that have identified CSFs and their receptors in placenta.[48] CSF-1 is greatly elevated in the uterus in pregnancy, being regulated by estrogens and progestagens. Whether they regulate placental and/or embryonic growth and development will, no doubt, be answered soon.

Immunological Traffic
at the Materno–Fetal Interface

Statements can be found to the effect that there is a *complete* separation of the maternal and fetal circulations. This might have been considered true on a fairly gross anatomical level, but it is now certain that there are important pathways for the travel of cells and molecules between the mother and the fetus. This section will consider immunologically relevant moities.

Antibody Passage Across the Placenta

Maternal IgG easily crosses the placenta from mother to fetus, but IgM does not. When only 2 immunoglobulin isotypes were recognized, it seemed to be obvious that this differential in transplacental movement was owing to the fact that the molecular "holes" in the membranes allowed the smaller IgG (160,000 mw) to go through, but blocked the exit of the very much larger IgM (900,000 mw). When IgA was discovered, and it was noted that although it had a mol wt of 160,000, very similar to that of IgG, yet it did not cross the placenta, this theory of free passage through a molecular sieve had to be abandoned. IgG has been found in fetal blood at the first time it was sampled (10 wk).[49] In later pregnancy, fetal levels of serum IgG were actually *higher than* in the mother,[50] indicating that IgG was being actively transported into the fetus against a concentration gradient, probably via coated vesicles on the syncytiotrophoblast.[51] Table 3 shows that the

Table 3
The Transfer of Maternal IgG from Mother to Fetus

Gestation (weeks)	Ratio: $\dfrac{\text{Fetal IgG}}{\text{Maternal IgG}}$
28	0.40
30	0.60
32	0.80
34	0.95
36	1.15
38	1.35
40	1.50

ratio of fetal to maternal serum IgG rises from 0.4 at 28 wk of gestation to 1.5 at 40 wk.[52] This transport of IgG involves the FcRγ in the placenta.[53] The placental FcRγ is one receptor with highest affinity for IgG1 and IgG3. It has lesser affinity for IgG2 and IgG4 and none for IgA or IgM.[54] Thus although IgM may indeed not cross the placenta because of its very large size, the failure of IgA (and IgD and IgE) to cross is owing to the lack of FcRs for those immunoglobulin isotypes.[51] All subclasses of IgG cross the placenta, and at term the fetal serum levels of IgG1, IgG2, IgG3, and IgG4 all exceed maternal levels.[52]

There is an exception, however, to the concept that all varieties of maternal IgG cross into the fetus. There is ample evidence that maternal antibodies to paternal HLA antigens on the fetus are adsorbed by the placenta. This finding (and others) gave rise to the idea of a *placental sink* for certain immunoglobulins. Anti-paternal HLA antibodies can be eluted from the placenta in almost all women who have these antibodies prior to delivery. The removal of these antibodies by the placenta is efficient, since they are not found in cord serum.[55,56] Furthermore, the titer of anti-HLA antibodies in the maternal serum begins to fall in the third trimester.[55,57] While some of this fall may be owing to hemodilution and transport into the fetus, the magnitude of the fall makes it appear that placental adsorption is also important. Data from the mouse show that Fab_2 anti-paternal antibodies as well as intact IgG are removed by placental tissue. As the Fab2 molecules lack the Fc portion, they are not taken up by the placental FcRs. This implies that indeed maternal antifetal HLA antibodies are removed by placental HLA itself. Since polymorphic HLA is not present on the trophoblast surface, either the anti-HLA antibodies are sponged up by the polymorphic HLA in the interstitium of the trophoblast or they adhere to HLA G on the trophoblast. At the present, there are no data pointing to one or the other of these possibilities.

Thus, the selectivity of immunoglobulin transport from mother to fetus has three aspects:

1. The facilitated passage of IgG across the placenta;
2. The failure to permit the passage of equally large immunoglobulins (e.g. IgA, IgD, IgE) into the fetus, and
3. The selective removal of anti-paternal HLA antibodies in the placental sink.

These three aspects of antibody metabolism are sufficiently different as to prompt questions about their possible survival value. The survival value of the maternal-to-fetal stream of IgG is to provide the fetus and neonate with antimicrobial antibodies until such time as the newborn infant can synthesize its own repertoire of immunoglobulin isotypes—IgG, IgA, IgM, IgD, and IgE.

On the other hand, we simply do not know if there is any benefit to the fetus in *not* receiving IgA, for instance, around the time of delivery. However, "nature" appears to have provided an alternate way to supply the fetus with just those major immunoglobulin isotypes that are not transported prior to birth. Breast milk is high in IgM and highest in IgA, whereas it is poor in IgG—the isotype least needed in the puerperium.[51]

Last, although we do not know if anti-paternal HLA antibodies would be injurious to the fetus, it is likely that they are, judging from data in which maternal anti-Rh antibodies or anti-platelet antibodies cause damage in the fetus. Thus the adsorption of anti-HLA antibodies by the placenta most likely has survival value. The situation may not be the same in the rodent where antipaternal antibodies can spill over into the fetus when the mother's antibody titer is high. However, these antibodies do not appear to cause damage, perhaps because they are noncytotoxic and do not fix complement.[58] We will see some interesting information in the next section about the reverse situation, i.e., the effect of anti-HLA antibodies in the mother on the survival of fetal leukocytes that have crossed the placenta.

Cell Traffic Across the Placenta

One can envision traffic of various kinds of cells between mother and fetus during pregnancy, while also recognizing that the placental disruption that occurs at delivery can provide additional opportunities for such traffic. In general, we will be concerned with materno–fetal traffic prior to delivery and will consider the passage of erythrocytes and lymphocytes in both directions.[59,60] We will also consider the transfer of trophoblast cells from embryo to mother.

Erythrocytes pass the placenta in both directions. *Fetus-to-mother* transfer increases as pregnancy advances. During the first trimester, 5% of pregnant women can be found to have fetal red cells in their circulation. The frequency of these cells is low, i.e., less than 1/50,000 erythrocytes. During the second and third trimesters, 20–40% of pregnant women have circulating fetal red cells, and the frequency is more than 1/50,000. As would be expected, more circulating fetal cells can be detected if there is no ABO incompatibility. However, this may not reflect any difference in erythrocyte traffic between ABO compatible vs ABO incompatible pregnancies, but only the fact that fetal cells, once they have crossed the placenta, will survive better in ABO compatible situations.

Mother-to-fetus transfer of erythrocytes is less well documented, as from 10 to 50% of pregnancies are reported to show the phenomenon. Furthermore, it is not clear when the bulk of this kind of transplacental traffic takes place nor what the magnitude may be.

Leukocytes also pass the placenta in both directions. Since granulocytes and monocytes have very short half-lives in the circulation, it is likely that most data in which the nature of the immigrant leukocyte is not specified reflect the passage of longer-lived lymphocytes. *Fetus-to-mother* transfer is said to occur frequently. Cultures of maternal blood with subsequent karyotypic analysis for male cells showed that fetal cells were present in the maternal circulation as early as 14 wk of gestation.[61] As fetal red cells were not seen, it is believed that leukotype transfer had occurred without "bleeding".[62] Similar results were obtained when flow cytometry was used to demonstrate the presence of HLA-2$^+$ leukocytes in the blood of mothers who were HLA-2$^-$ but carried HLA-2$^+$ fetuses.[63] Seven of 11 women carrying male fetuses had circulating leukocytes with a Y chromosome. These fetal cells comprised about 0.1–0.5% of the circulating lymphocytes and were seen as early as 4 months of gestation, which was the earliest time tested.[64] It is instructive but not surprising that when cytotoxic antipaternal HLA antibodies were present in the maternal circulation, it was difficult or impossible to detect fetal cells.[64] Presumably they were either lysed or opsonized and removed in the maternal reticulo-endothelial system, although there is some evidence that there may be masking of the HLA antigens on the persisting fetal cells in the maternal blood.[65] This fact also gives us information as to whether there is a benefit to the fetus in *not* having maternal anti-paternal HLA antibodies cross the placenta. If these antibodies, when present in the maternal circulation, do not permit the survival of immigrant fetal cells, it is more than likely that they would aid in the destruction of the fetus' own circulating cells should these antibodies cross into the embryo.

Mother-to-fetus transfer of leukocytes also occurs but it understandably more difficult to show. Maternal PBL labeled in vitro with atabrine and reinfused near the time of delivery were found in the newborn blood.[66] Whether such mother-to-fetus lymphoid deportation occurs earlier in pregnancy (where it might be more critical to materno–fetal development) is not clear.[60] The consequences of maternal-to-fetal leukocyte transfer, in terms of possible graft-vs-host disease, will be discussed later (Chapter 5).

The passage of trophoblast cells from embryo to mother is called *trophoblast deportation.* An early study of 220 pregnancies reported that there was morphological evidence for trophoblast embolization in 44% of the cases. The incidence of such emboli increased as pregnancy advanced, and was greatest in the perinatal period. However, these results were derived from postmortem analyses. The pregnancies or their finales were obviously not normal, and there were many cases of eclampsia, hemorrhage, and shock.[67] As the study of HLA antigens was in its infancy, the authors did not consider possible immunological consequences of trophoblast deportation. Further studies have brought current technology to bear on this question. Another approach used a monoclonal antibody (H315) that recognized a choriocarcinoma line and normal syncytiotrophoblast but not PBL to detect circulating trophoblast cells in retroplacental blood.[68] Several kinds of cells or fragments were seen. When this approach was applied to peripheral blood in pregnancy, circulating trophoblastic cells were seen in up to 80% at some time in pregnancy. Two of 5 patients studied as early as the first 10 weeks of gestation had circulating trophoblastic cells. In all cases, the frequency was less than 10/1,000 peripheral blood nucleated cells. Using newer techniques, maternal blood from 12 first-trimester and 1 third-trimester pregnancies was studied. Putative deported trophoblast cells were isolated by their affinity for trophoblast-specific antibodies. The DNA from these few cells was isolated and amplified by the polymerase chain reaction (PCR), a very sensitive method for detecting small amounts of specific DNA. The amplified material was probed for the presence of male-specific DNA sequences. The correct fetal sex assignment was made in 12/13 cases. The results indicated that fetal trophoblast cells were present in maternal blood in almost every first trimester. Again, the time of the first transplacental traffic and the number and lifespan of the deported cells was not specified.

The consequences of trophoblast deportation are not known. To a great degree, the fate of the cells in the mother depend on what alloantigens are expressed and how the maternal immune system responds to them. If the trophoblast cells only exhibit the nonpolymorphic HLA-G, it is not likely that any immune recognition will occur. If there is Rh(D) or polymorphic HLA from interstitial trophoblast tissue, the cells will be disposed of rapidly if the mother has antibodies to these alloantigens. If she does not, it is possible that some sort of allosensitization may occur. However, there is also the intriguing possibility that tolerance rather than sensitization may develop in the mother.

Summary

1. Immunologic events may occur at the physical materno–fetal interface where the trophoblast meets maternal tissue, or by exchange of fetal and maternal materials as they cross the placenta.
2. A principal point of inquiry has been into the question of major histocompatibility complex (MHC) antigen expression by the fetal trophoblast.
   a. Conventional polymorphic HLA antigens are not expressed at the materno–fetal interface.
   b. Instead, a truncated form of HLA class I molecule called HLA-G is present on the nonvillous and villous trophoblast. It shows limited, if any, polymorphism, and is not up-regulated by IFN-γ.
3. Other antigenic systems are also expressed on the trophoblast. These include a trophoblast–leukocyte cross-reacting (TLX) system, erythrocyte blood-group antigens, alkaline phosphatase, immunoglobulin Fc receptors, and NK target structures. The significance of any of these systems in materno–fetal alloreactivity is not certain.

4. Immunoglobulin passage occurs across the materno–fetal barrier.

a. Maternal IgG crosses the placenta by facilitated transport; however, anti-HLA antibodies, even if IgG, are absorbed in the "placental sink" and do not reach the fetus.

5. Cellular traffic occurs in both directions.

a. Fetal erythrocytes may sensitize the mother, e.g., to Rh and other antigens.

b. Trophoblast cells frequently cross into the maternal circulation, i.e., "trophoblast deportation."

c. Maternal lymphocytes may reach the fetus and, in rare circumstances, be responsible for graft-vs-host phenomena.

References

1. Benirschke K, Kaufmann P: *Pathology of the Human Placenta*, New York, Springer-Verlag; 1991.
2. Loke YW, Butterworth BH: Heterogeneity of human trophoblast populations, in Wegmann TG, Gill III TJ (eds): *Immunoregulation and Fetal Survival*. New York, Oxford University Press; 1987: 197–209.
3. Simmons RL, Russell PS: Antigenicity of mouse trophoblast. *Ann N Y Acad Sci* 1962; 99: 717–732.
4. Faulk WP, Temple A: Distribution of β_2-microglobulin and HLA in chorionic villi of human placentae. *Nature* 1976; 262: 799–802.
5. Sutton L, Mason DY, Redman CWG: HLA-DR positive cells in the human placenta. *Immunology* 1983; 49: 103–112.
6. Wells M, Bulmer JN: The human placental bed: Histology, immunochemistry and pathology. *Histopathology* 1988; 13: 483–498.
7. Redman C, McMichael AJ, Stirrat GM, et al: Class I MHC antigens on human extravillous trophoblast. *Immunology* 1984; 52: 457–468.
8. Ellis S: HLA G: At the interface. *Am J Reprod Immunol* 1990; 23: 84–86.
9. Kovats S, Main EK, Librach C, Stubblebine M, Fisher SJ, DeMars R: A class I antigen, HLA-G, expressed in human trophoblasts. *Science* 1990; 248: 220–223.

10. Ellis SA, Palmer MS, McMichael AJ: Human trophoblast and the choriocarcinoma cell line BeWo express a truncated HLA class I molecule. *J Immunol* 1990; 144: 731–735.

11. Kovats S, Librach C, Fisch P, et al.: Expression and possible function of the HLA-G alpha chain in human cytotrophoblasts, in Chaouat G, Mowbray J (eds): *Cellular and Molecular Biology of the Materno-Fetal Relationship.* INSERM/J. Libbey Eurotext, Ltd.; 1991: 21–29.

12. Harris HW, Gill IV TJ: Expression of class I transplantation antigens. *Transplantation* 1986; 42: 109–117.

13. Desoye G, Dohr GA, Ziegler A: Biology of disease: Expression of human major histocompatibility antigens on germ cells and early preimplantation of embryos. *Lab Invest* 1991; 64: 306–312.

14. Desoye G, Dohr GA, Motter W, et al: Lack of HLA class I and class II antigens on human preimplantation embryos. *J Immunol* 1988; 140: 4157–4159.

15. Hunt JS, Yelavarthi KK, Yangi Y, et al: Class I major histo-compatibility genes in trophoblast cells: Studies on expression, regulation and function, in Chaouat G, Mowbray J (eds): *Cellular and Molecular Biology of the Materno-Fetal Relationship.* INSERM/J. Libbey Eurotext, Ltd.; 1991: 51–59.

16. Yelavarthi KK, Fishback JL, Hunt JS: Analysis of HLA-G mRNA in human placental and extraplacental membrane cells by in situ hybridization. *J Immunol* 1991; 146: 2847–2854.

17. Ijzermans JNM, Marquet RL: Interferon-gamma: A review. *Immunobiology* 1989; 179: 456–473.

18. Hunt JS, Andrews GK, Wood GW: Normal trophoblasts resist induction of class I HLA. *J Immunol* 1987; 138: 2481–2487.

19. Head JR, Drake BL, Zuckerman FA: MHC antigens on tropho-blast and their regulations: Implications in the maternal-fetal relationship. *Am J Reprod Immunol* 1987; 15: 12–18.

20. Faulk WP, Temple A, Lovins RE, et al: Antigens of human trophoblasts: A working hypothesis for their role in normal and abnormal pregnancies. *Proc Natl Acad Sci USA* 1978; 75: 1947–1951.

21. Rocklin RE, Kitzmiller JL, Carpenter CB, et al: Maternal-fetal relation: Absence of an immunologic blocking factor from the serum of women with chronic abortions. *N Engl J Med* 1976; 295: 1209–1213.

22. McIntyre JA, Faulk WP: Allotypic trophoblast-lymphocyte cross-reactive (TLX) cell surface antigens. *Hum Immunol* 1982; 4: 27–35.

23. McIntyre JA, Faulk WP, Verhulst SJ, et al: Human trophoblast lymphocyte cross-reactive (TLX) antigens define a new alloantigen system. *Science* 1983; 222: 1135–1137.

24. Stern PL, Beresford N, Thompson S, et al: Characterization of the human trophoblast-leukocyte common antigen molecules defined by a monoclonal antibody. *J Immunol* 1986; 137: 1604–1609.

25. Torry DS, Faulk WP, McIntyre JA: Regulation of immunity to extraembryonic antigens in human pregnancy. *Am J Reprod Immunol* 1989; 21: 76–81.

26. MacLeod AM, Stewart KN, Catto GRD, et al: Immunological studies of trophoblast antigens: No evidence for human leucocyte antigen (HLA) linkage. *Am J Reprod Immunol* 1989; 19: 11–16.

27. Kim IC: Isolation and identification of trophoblast lymphocyte cross-reactive (TLX) antigens from human lymphocytes. *J Biol Chem* 1989; 264: 9780–9784.

28. McIntyre JA: In search of trophoblast-lymphocyte crossreactive (TLX) antigens. *Am J Reprod Immunol Microbiol* 1988; 17: 100–110.

29. Hsi BBL, Fenichel P, Milesi-Fluet C, et al: Expression of complementary regulatory proteins on human gametes and trophoblast, in Chaouat G, Mowbray J (eds): *Cellular and Molecular Biology of the Materno-Fetal Relationship*. INSERM/ J. Libbey Eurotext, Ltd.; 1991: 3–11.

30. Beer AE: Immunologic aspects of normal pregnancy and recurrent spontaneous abortion. *Semin Reprod Endocrinol* 1988; 6: 163–180.

31. David-Watine B: Expression of major histocompatibility antigens on fetal and placental cells, in Chaouat G (ed): *The Immunology of the Fetus*. Boca Raton, FL, CRC Press, Inc.; 1990: 53–74.

32. Goto S, Nishi H, Tomoda Y: Blood group Rh-D factor in human trophoblast determined by immunofluorescent method. *Am J Obstet Gynecol* 1980; 137: 707–712.

33. Johnson PM, Risk JM, Bulmer JN, et al.: Antigen expression at human maternofetal interfaces, in Wegmann TG, Gill III TJ (eds): *Immunoregulation and Fetal Survival*. New York, Oxford University Press; 1987: 181–196.

34. Faulk WP, Hunt JS: Human placentae: View from an immunological bias. *Am J Reprod Immunol* 1989; 21: 108–113.

35. Saji F, Kameda T, Koyama M, et al: Impaired susceptibility of human trophoblast to MHC nonrestricted killer cells: Implication in the maternal-fetal relationship. *Am J Reprod Immunol* 1989; 19: 108–113.
36. Bulmer JN, Longfellow M, Ritson A: Leukocytes and resident blood cells in endometrium. *Ann N Y Acad Sci* 1991; 221: 57–68.
37. Bulmer JN, Johnson PM: The T lymphocyte population in first trimester human decidua does not express the interleukin-2 receptor. *Immunology* 1986; 58: 685–687.
38. Ferenczy A, Bergeron C: Histology of the human endometrium: From birth to senescence. *Ann NY Acad Sci* 1991; 622: 6–27.
39. King A, Loke YW: On the nature and function of human uterine granular lymphocytes. *Immunol Today* 1991; 12: 432–435.
40. Vaquer S, de la Hera A, Jorda J, et al: Diminished natural killer activity in pregnancy: Modulation by interleukin 2 and interferon gamma. *Scand J Immunol* 1987; 26: 691–698.
41. Ferry BL, Starkey PM, Sargent IL, et al: Cell populations in the human early pregnancy decidua: Natural killer activity and response to interleukin-2 CD56-positive large granular lymphocytes. *Immunology* 1990; 70: 446–452.
42. Pace D, Morrison L, Bulmer JN: Proliferative activity in endometrial stromal granulocytes throughout menstrual cycle and early pregnancy. *J Clin Pathol* 1989; 42: 35–39.
43. King A, Loke YW: Uterine large granular lymphocytes: A possible role in embryonic implantation? *Am J Obstet Gynecol* 1990; 162: 308–310.
44. Manaseki S, Searle RF: Natural killer (NK) cell activity of first trimester human decidua. *Cell Immunol* 1989; 121: 166–173.
45. Toder V, Shomer B: The role of lymphokines in pregnancy. *Immunol Allergy Clinics N Am* 1990; 10: 65–77.
46. Chin TW, Ank BJ, Strom SR, et al.: Enhanced interferon production and lymphokine-activated cytotoxicity of human placental cells. *Cell Immunol* 1988; 113: 1–9.
47. Athanassakis I, Bleackley RC, Paetkau V, et al: The immuno-stimulatory effect of T cells and T cell lymphokines on murine fetally derived placental cells. *J Immunol* 1987; 138: 37–44.
48. Pollard JW, Pampfer S, Arceci RJ: Class III tyrosine kinase receptors at the maternal-fetal interface, in Chaouat G, Mowbray

J (eds): *Cellular and Molecular Biology of the Materno-Fetal Relationship*. INSERM/J. Libbey Eurotext, Ltd.; 1991: 81–89.

49. Chandra RK: Levels of IgG subclasses, IgA, IgM and tetanus antitoxin in paired maternal and foetal sera: Findings in healthy pregnancy and placental insufficiency, in Hemmings WA (ed): *Maternofoetal Transmission of Immunoglobulins*. London, Cambridge University Press; 1976: 77–90.

50. Kohler PF, Farr RS: Elevation of cord over maternal IgG immunoglobulin: Evidence for an active placental IgG transport. *Nature* 1966; 210: 1070.

51. Nervard CHF, Gaunt M, Ockleford CD: The transfer of passive and active immunity, in Chaouat G (ed): *The Immunology of the Fetus*. Baco Raton, CRC Press, Inc.; 1990: 193–214.

52. Pitcher-Wilmott RW, Hindocha P, Wood CBS: The placental transfer of immunoglobulin and subclasses in human pregnancy. *Clin Exp Immunol* 1980; 41: 303–308.

53. Johnson PM, Trenchev P, Faulk PW: Immunological studies of human placentae binding of complexed immunoglobulin by stromal endothelial cells. *Clin Exp Immunol* 1975; 22: 133–138.

54. McNabb T, Koh TY, Dorrington KJ, et al: Structure and function of immunoglobulin domains. V. Binding of immunoglobulin G and fragments to placental membrane preparations. *J Immunol* 1976; 117: 882–888.

55. Doughty RW, Gelsthorpe K: An initial investigation of lymphocyte antibody activity through pregnancy and in eluates prepared from placental material. *Tissue Antigens* 1972; 4: 291–298.

56. Jeannet M, Werner C, Ramirez E, et al: Anti-HLA, anti-human "Ia-like" and MLC blocking activity of human placental IgG. T*ransplant Proc* 1977; IX: 1417–1422.

57. Doughty RW, Gelsthorpe K: Some parameters of lymphocyte antibody activity through pregnancy and further eluates of placental material. *Tissue Antigens* 1976; 8: 43–48.

58. Bell SC, Billington WD: Anti-fetal allo-antibody in the pregnant female. *Immunol Rev* 1983; 75: 5–30.

59. Shroder J: Transplacental passage of blood cells. *J Med Genet* 1975; 12: 230–242.

60. Gill III TJ: Chimerism in humans. *Transplant Proc* 1977; 9: 1423–1431.

61. Walkanowska J, Conte FA, Grumbach MM: Practical and theoretical implications of fetal/maternal lymphocyte transfer. *Lancet* 1969; i: 1119–1122.

62. Zilliacus R, de la Chapelle A, Schroder J, et al: Transplacental passage of foetal blood cells. *Scand J Haematol* 1975; 15: 333–338.

63. Herzenberg LA, Bianchi DW, Schroder J, et al: Fetal cells in the blood of pregnant women: Detection and enrichment by fluorescence-activated cell sorting. *Proc Natl Acad Sci USA* 1979; 76: 1453–1450.

64. Schroder J, de la Chapelle A: Fetal lymphocytes in the maternal blood. *Blood* 1972; 39: 153–162.

65. Tilikainen A, Schroder J, de la Chapelle A: Fetal leukocytes in the maternal circulation after delivery. II. Masking of HL-A antigens. *Transplantation* 1974; 17: 355–360.

66. Desai RG, Creger WP: Materofetal passage of leukocytes and platelets in man. *Blood* 1963; 21: 665–673.

67. Attwood HD, Park WW: Embolism to the lungs by trophoblast. *J Obstet Gynaecol Br Commonw* 1961; 68: 611–617.

68. Covone A, Mutton ED, Johnson PM, et al: Trophoblast cells in peripheral blood from pregnant women. *Lancet* 1984; 2: 841–843.

Chapter 3

Maternal Immunocompetence During Pregnancy

One of the standard explanations for the survival of the fetal allograft is that there is a general depression of the mother's immune response during pregnancy. One author has claimed that there is a "pregnancy-associated immune deficiency syndrome."[1] This chapter will explore the data that suggest that there are modifications of immune competence associated with pregnancy. Such modifications might be systemic or local (or both). Finally, we will explore that most interesting question: Is the uterus an immunologically privileged site?

The Systemic Immune Response in Pregnancy

Resistance to Infectious Disease as an Indication of Maternal Immunocompetence

Abundant experimental and clinical data indicate that an increased susceptibility to infection is a consequence of impaired immunocompetence. Indeed, an excessive incidence or severity of infections is a clinical clue that may lead the physician to suspect immunological impairment.

Whether there is a pregnancy-associated decrease in resistance to infectious disease is a complex question. In a classic and comprehensive review,[2] Brabin begins by saying that "it is generally agreed that a woman is at greater risk of infection when pregnant." Immediately, however, one must ask questions such as: Which infections are most implicated? When in pregnancy is resistance lowered? What is the primary type of immunological defense against the infection in question? Are there different risks for relapse, reactivation, or reinfection? What is the effect of parity? Are pregnant women more exposed to the microbe in question than nonpregnant women? What is the role of possible pregnancy-associated malnutrition in apparent decreased resistance to infection? What is the role of antimicrobial therapy?

Almost none of these questions has been answered definitely and comprehensively, but there are some interesting data. There is evidence that there is an increase in the clinical severity of certain newly-acquired infections when they occur in pregnancy. These include: viral infections—hepatitis, variola, and influenza, but not varicella (in the absence of pneumonia); bacterial infections—cholera, scarlet fever, gonorrhea, and typhoid; and at least one fungal disease, namely, coccidioidomycosis.[1] In coccidioidomycosis, there is an increased risk to both mother and fetus, but this is most striking in the second and third trimesters.[3] Leprosy also tends to be more severe in late pregnancy, whereas there is an increased incidence of listeriosis an pregnancy in general.[4]

Reactivation of latent infections in "immune" women during pregnancy has been seen with herpes viruses, such as cytomegalovirus and Epstein-Barr virus.[5] There is little definitive information available for genital herpes or viral hepatitis.

Tuberculosis represents an interesting situation. Despite the widely held opinion that pregnancy has a deleterious effect on tuberculosis, there are papers stating that it has *no* effect. There are even some statements indicating that pregnancy is beneficial for tuberculosis! A comprehensive review by Hedvall[6] concludes that leaving aside the protection afforded by specific chemotherapy most current opinions indicate that pregnancy does not present a special risk for tuberculosis.

Immune Responses to Conventional Antigens in Pregnancy

One method of assessing the immunocompetence of the pregnant woman is to measure either her response to new antigens, or her expression of immunity to previously encountered antigens (recall). A careful prospective study showed that the serum antibody responses of women given influenza vaccine in the first, second, or third trimester were no different from the responses seen in similarly immunized nonpregnant women.[7] Several groups have asked whether pregnancy produces changes in the serum levels of autoantibodies in women with autoimmune syndromes. In many (but not all) patients, titers of antithyroglobulin and antimicrosomal antibodies fell as pregnancy progressed in women with autoimmune thyroid disease.[8] The same phenomenon was seen with insulin-binding antibodies in pregnant diabetics.[9] In neither situation was hemodilution believed to be responsible, yet the cause of the fall in antibody titers is unexplained.

Those investigators who have measured the elicitation of delayed-type hypersensitivity (DTH) by means of conventional tuberculin-type recall skin tests have usually found no changes in pregnancy.[10] Another study, however, found only minor degrees of inhibition of established DTH in pregnancy.[11] Nevertheless, the changes found hardly seem sufficient to account for either increases in certain infections or for any nonreactivity toward the fetus.[4]

The "Immunologic Machinery" in Pregnancy

The methods available to study the various cellular and humoral elements of the immune system have been used to assess these elements during pregnancy, It is generally agreed that maternal serum IgG falls as pregnancy progresses. Part of this fall may be caused by hemodilution, although the stability of serum IgA and IgM levels argues strongly that hemodilution cannot be the whole answer. IgG levels may also decrease because this protein is actively transported across the placenta to the fetus, whereas IgA and IgM are not (Chapter 2). Last, Fc receptors for IgG may remove some maternal immunoglobulin in the "placental sink."

It is widely believed that the numbers of circulating lymphocytes, as well as the numbers and ratios of T helpers/T suppressors and T/B cells may reflect overall immunocompetence. Certainly the devastation that HIV infection produces in the CD4$^+$ T cell population does a great deal to explain the immunosuppression seen in AIDS. In pregnancy, early studies appeared to show that there was an increase in the percentage of B cells and a decrease in the percentage of T cells during the first 22 weeks of pregnancy.[12] Subsequent studies, however, using improved methods for T and B cell enumeration failed to support the earlier findings.[13-15] An occasional report shows a decrease in CD4$^+$ cells in early pregnancy,[16] but still other data have not demonstrated significant changes in T cells or T cell subsets during the 1st, 2nd, and 3rd trimesters.[17] A prospective study did show decreases in T cell numbers and percentages in the second and third trimesters, but the changes, although statistically significant, did not convince the investigators that they were biologically relevant to any putative immunodeficiency of pregnancy.[18] In short, most investigators believe that changes in peripheral blood lymphocyte populations are not very important in pregnancy.[19]

Functional studies of lymphocyte responses in vitro give varying results. One group found that PHA responses dipped as pregnancy advanced,[20] but another group found no change.[21] The latter investigation also described lymphocyte proliferative responses to PPD in pregnancy women who were tuberculin positive. The antigen-driven response was normal in the first and second trimesters, but it dipped at 36 weeks and was very low immediately postpartum. Interestingly, it became normal 4 weeks after delivery. Such results argue for a decrease in CMI late in pregnancy, but would not be pertinent to maternal immunocompetence during the crucial early weeks.

Little work has been done to evaluate systematically the nonspecific elements of the inflammatory response. One intriguing paper shows that polymorphonuclear leukocyte chemotaxis is significantly depressed in the second and third trimesters, but not in the first three months.[22] Another group has shown that natural killer (NK) activity is defective in the blood of pregnant women. The investigators believe that this is owing to impaired maturation of NK precursors, and that this defect can be overcome (at least in vitro) by additional IL-2.[23] This interesting approach supports other data indicating that the IL-2 system may not function normally in pregnancy.

Local Immune Responses in the Uterus

The female genitourinary tract can be considered to be a part of the mucosal immune system. As such, one may expect it to be able to mount local immune responses to local antigens of various kinds, microbial or nonmicrobial. Data on this point are understandably sparse in the human. Ogra found that immunization via the genital tract with poliovirus led to local antibody formation.[24] The predominating isotype of the antibody produced depended on the route of immunization. Intrauterine antigen provoked local IgG responses. Intravaginal immunization led to both IgA and IgG production with IgA predominating. These isotype differences indicate a degree of immunological specialization within the genital mucosal immune system.[25]

If mucosal elements of the immune system in the uterus were responding to paternal antigens in the fetus, one might expect to see changes in the draining parauterine lymph nodes. Experiments in mice have shown that the parauterine nodes are larger during pregnancies between allogeneic parents (allopregnancies) when compared with the same nodes in pregnancies between parents that are identical at the major histocompatibility loci (synpregnancies).[26] (Such data might lead one to expect that the processes within the nodes in allopregnancies are anti-MHC, but it is possible that they represent mechanisms *inhibiting* allorecognition and alloresponses [*see* section on suppressor mechanisms].) However, other work using more defined strains of mice that differ *only* at the MHC and not at loci coding for the many minor histocompatibility antigens, did not find any significant differences in lymph node, placental, or fetal weights.[27] The ability to use carefully controlled genetic combinations in mice make this an attractive area of investigation. The outcome of such work is not always what was anticipated. It was found that T cell responses to mitogens were decreased in lymph nodes draining the uterus during pregnancy, but it was decreased equally in allogeneic and syngeneic pregnancies.[28] This result, at least in the murine system, does not contribute strength to the concept of important maternal–fetal allorecognition.

There are only occasional references that include information on parauterine responses in human pregnancy. One group mentioned that parauterine lymph nodes are *smaller* in pregnancy than in the nongravid condition.[20] Since human pregnancies are allopregnancies, this is a paradoxical result. This entire subject needs more detailed investigation.

Immunoregulation in the Pregnant Woman

Clearly, all immune responses are regulated as to their type, (e.g., humoral vs cellular), magnitude, duration, and so forth, and a great deal of current immunologic research is trained on the various mechanisms responsible for such regulation. Since pregnancy brings with it a variety of cellular and humoral changes not seen in nongravidae, it is pertinent to ask what immunoregulatory effects these changes might entail. This section will discuss pregnancy-associated hormones and proteins (Table 1) as well as suppressor processes.

Table 1
Hormones and Proteins Associated with Pregnancy[32,33]

I. Steroid hormones
corticosteroids
progesterone
estrogens
II. Alphafetoprotein
III. Trophoblast-derived hormones and proteins
human chorionic gonadotrophin
pregnancy-associated plasma proteins (PAPP)
PAPP-A
PAPP-B
PAPP-C (SP-1)
PAPP-D (human placental lactogen)
pregnancy zone protein (PZP) (SP-3)
SP-2

Hormones and Proteins Associated with Pregnancy

Enormous changes occur in the hormonal milieu in pregnancy. These changes involve steroid hormones, alphafetoprotein, and trophoblast-derived hormones.

Glucocorticosteroids (corticosteroids) are known modulators of immune responses, and their metabolism is altered in pregnancy. Indeed, the amelioration of rheumatoid arthritis, which often occurs in pregnancy, was one of the two clinical "pearls" that led Hench and colleagues to the long search that resulted in the identification of compound E as a new and potent anti-inflammatory drug.[29] (Paradoxically, it is still not clear exactly what the mechanism is by which pregnancy improves rheumatoid arthritis, *see* Chapter 5.) Among animals, rodents are very susceptible to exogenous corticosteroids, and both cellular and humoral responses are not difficult to inhibit with these drugs. Humans are more resistant to the immunosuppressive effects of corticosteroids,[30] yet large doses are clinically effective in preventing allograft rejection and in the treatment of autoimmune syndromes.[31] Blood levels of free (active) corticosteroids are increased in pregnancy, but there is little evidence that such concentrations produce a significant systemic immunosuppressive effect in the mother.[32] Whether there are local intraplacental effects not seen elsewhere in the pregnant state remains unclear.

Sex hormones are known to affect the immune system, and *progesterone* is greatly elevated in the plasma of pregnant women beginning in the first trimester. It is first produced by the corpus luteum and later by the placenta itself. Maternal plasma levels rise from 2 to 12 to 17 µg/mL at the 9th, the 35th, and the 40th week, respectively.[33] A level of 5 µg/mL has been measured in placental blood, and Clemons et al. have studied the effect of this amount of progesterone on the MLR in humans.[34] There was a 25% reduction in the MLR when progesterone was present for the entire 120-h culture period. Thus, progesterone at concentrations reached in late (but not early) pregnancy may indeed modestly inhibit reactions of the cell-mediated variety. *Estrogens* are not present in such high concentrations in pregnancy, nor do they have immunosuppressive abilities comparable to progesterone.

Alphafetoprotein (AFP) was first obtained from the amniotic fluid of mice, and Murgita and Tomasi showed that it inhibited both mitogen stimulation and the MLR in that species.[35] There have been, however, a number of problems in determining whether AFP is a pertinent pregnancy-associated immunoregulatory substance. Earlier preparations were purified by electrophoresis, but analysis was difficult because there were both inhibitory and stimulatory factors in the material. Furthermore, although AFP inhibited immune processes in vivo and in vitro in the mouse, it did not do so in the rat. Human amniotic fluid preparations containing AFP do inhibit mitogen responses of human peripheral blood leukocytes, but the degree of suppression does not correlate with the AFP content of the fluid.[36] Thus, the importance of AFP as a relevant immunosuppressive protein in humans is doubtful. Another substance that has also been reported to have suppressive activities, namely early pregnancy factor (EPF) is discussed below.

Human chorionic gonadotropin (hCG) plasma levels begin to rise extremely soon after conception. They plateau during the first trimester before declining. Early studies suggested that hCG may be a powerful immunosuppressant, but later work indicated that the inhibitory activity was the result of a contaminating substance.[32,33,37] There are a number of *Pregnancy-Associated Plasma Proteins* (PAPPs) that have been described by many workers under a variety of names[32,33] (Table 1). The terminology is confusing. For instance, PAPP-C has also been called Schwangerschafts protein-1, or SP-1. Proteins like this one are often not specific for pregnancy, yet their concentrations in the serum rise as pregnancy continues. These substances hold some interest because they have been shown to inhibit human leukocyte function in vitro, generally affecting either mitogen stimulation or the MLR.[32,33] However, the general state of uncertainty in this area is exemplified by the results of Johannsen et al.[38] They found that although the MLR was inhibited by α-2 macroglobulin, there was also MLR inhibition by antibodies to α-2 macroglobulin. Thus, although these proteins are not polymorphic, and hence do not function as pregnancy antigens, they may play a role, particularly in the decidua, in downregulating immune reactivity.

Suppressor Mechanisms in Pregnancy

Systemic Immunosuppression in Pregnancy

Suppressor phenomena that regulate the immune response have been studied for a number of years (Chapter 1). Antigen-specific and antigen-nonspecific downregulation of both the cellular and humoral arms of the immune response can be seen in vivo and in vitro, in human and animal experiments. What is not always clear is what the precise nature of these mechanisms may be. The same questions may be raised about pregnancy-associated suppressor effects, but there are indications that the phenomena observed may be relevant to pregnancy immunology.

An important paper was published by Kasakura in 1971.[39] He studied the effect of *pregnancy plasma* on two-way MLRs. Pregnancy plasma significantly inhibited MLRs between the mother's PBL and her newborn's PBL, and also inhibited MLRs between unrelated pairs of PBL. Serum was taken at intervals between twelve weeks of pregnancy and delivery; the later in pregnancy, the more inhibitory the plasma. Fetal plasma showed somewhat different results, as it suppressed MLRs between mother and newborn but did not inhibit MLRs between unrelated subjects. This kind of experiment is a prototype for a large number of studies that look at immunomodulatory pathways peculiar to pregnancy. It is not clear whether any or all of the hormones or pregnancy-associated proteins mentioned above are responsible for the inhibitory properties of pregnancy serum. In fact, we know neither the nature nor the mechanism of the inhibitory properties of pregnancy plasma.

More recent experiments are beginning to focus on cytokines as possible mediators of pregnancy-associated immunoregulation. The suppressive effects of pregnancy serum on MLRs may be caused by an inhibition of IL-2 production,[40,41] but the origin of this effect awaits clarification.

There was some interest in a material called *early pregnancy factor* (EPF), first described in 1974. It was detected in the serum within hours of implantation but its measurement depended on a clumsy and difficult cellular rosette inhibition test.[42] Later reviews of the subject expressed a "healthy scepticism" about the function (and nature) of EPF,[43] but research in this area has remained productive in some hands.[44]

It is logical to ask whether suppressor cells may be present in pregnancy. As with suppressor cell research in general, the experiments often leave much to be desired. Often, the experiment involves MLR and/or CTL reactions involving maternal responders and newborn or paternal stimulators. What must be remembered is that paternal stimulators are generally completely allogeneic to the mother, whereas offspring cells are haploidentical. Haploidentical stimulators in general provoke only half the MLR when compared with completely allogeneic cells.[45]

It has been reported that selected parous women generate CTLs in MLRs with their husbands' cells as stimulators.[46] The paper lacked controls, and another group failed to find CTLs in this situation.[47] Suppressor activity has been seen in some maternal–paternal MLR combinations[48] and has been ascribed to T cells.[47] In one unusual family, a woman had T suppressor cells in her blood 9 years after the birth of her 10th child. She was homozygous at HLA-B and -DR and her husband was homozygous for different -B and -DR antigens. This rare situation was useful in determining the specificity of her T suppressors.[49]

Some data have shown that pregnancy blood contains "short-lived suppressor cell" (SLSC) activity.[50] In this kind of study, mitogenic responses to suboptimal doses of Con A are higher after PBL are first cultured alone for 24 h when compared to the responses of "fresh" PBL, where the mitogen is added on the first day. Presumably, some suppressor cell or activity is lost in the early culture period. The nature of the suppressor cell or activity is not known.

Local Immunosuppression in Pregnancy

Suppressive influences have been seen in the uterine environment. Even in the nonparous state, there is evidence for inhibitory factors. Human endometrium was cultured and the supernatants assayed for the ability to inhibit nonspecific mitogen responses and MLRs between random peripheral blood leukocytes. Inhibitory activity was present in supernatants from both proliferative and secretory phases but was greater with secretory endometrium.[51] Early gestational human decidua is also capable of suppressing lymphocyte alloreactivity in vitro nonspecifically.[52,53] The effects seem to center around decreased IL-2 and IL-2R production. Prostaglandins may be partly responsible as indomethacin (in high doses) reverses the inhibitors effect. The cells responsible for making the inhibitory substance(s) were not identified, but the relations between the inhibitory activity and the menstrual phases bring to mind the similar patterns of the increasing mitotic activity of K cells.[54] This raises the possibility that K cells may be responsible for the inhibitory properties of human endometrial cultures.

Less focused experiments have shown that cultures of human placentas, albeit at term, develop supernatants able to inhibit murine and human T cell function, i.e., MLRs and the generation of cytotoxic T cells (CTLs). This inhibition is reversed in part by adding IL-2.[55] Even at the blastocyst stage, human embryos can elaborate a supernatant that will suppress an MLR but not a nonspecific mitogen response.[56] Further insight into the mechanisms of placental immunosuppression comes from work showing that human decidual cells block allogeneic MLRs by secreting PGE-2, which, in turn, blocked the generation of IL-2 and IL-2 receptors.[57] Indomethacin or anti-PGE-2 not only reversed these inhibitions but augmented the appearance of cells cytotoxic for trophoblast targets. The implication is clear: Cells resembling lymphokine-activated killer (LAK) cells are potentially present in the decidua and may become injurious unless their generation and/or activity are frustrated by a lack of IL-2 production. Conversely, a process that promotes extra IL-2 production in the decidua (infection, for example?) might have deleterious effects by upregulating LAK activity.

More pertinent to the immunological paradox of pregnancy are the findings of Daya and Clark.[58–61] They found small lymphocytes in 13–16-week human placentas that suppress the mitogenic response of PBL to concanavalin A. (Whether these are the same as the suppressor cells described in[62] is not known.) They also found large lymphocyte-like suppressor cells in nonpregnant luteal phase endometrium but not in proliferative endometrium. The small cells released suppressive supernatants that blocked IL-2 activity. The large suppressor cells would also release a suppressor supernatant if cocultured with syncytiotrophoblast (but some small lymphocytes needed to be present as well). This group points out that there are at least 3 types of cells that express suppressor activity in vitro:

1. A trophoblast-independent stromal suppressor cell that inhibits T cell function via the production of PGE-2;
2. A trophoblast-dependent small cell that so far has an Fc receptor as its only marker. This cell makes soluble factor(s) that block the response of T and NK cells to IL-2; and
3. A large CD8⁺ cell that is hormone-dependent in that it is seen only in the luteal phase of the menstrual cycle and in pregnancy.[61]

Fetal Immunosuppression

Although the fetus has a degree of immunocompetence, it is not equal to that seen in the mature person. Are there any suppressor influences? Human cord blood lymphocytes inhibit both syngeneic and allogeneic T cell functions in vitro (reviewed in[62]). These cells can be demonstrated as early as the 8th week of pregnancy in the fetal liver. Many data indicate that these are CD4⁺ cells, but not all workers agree as some have found suppressive activity associated with CD8⁺ cells. The mechanism of inhibition has not been worked out, but prostaglandin E2 may be responsible at least in part because a significant amount of the inhibitory activity is blocked by indomethacin.

To make a generalization, one can say that there are tantalizing hints that suppressor activity can be found in pregnancy blood, in the decidua, and in cord blood. The methodologies in some of the reported studies are often less than optimal. Nevertheless, there are enough hints to suggest that immunologically-mediated reactions at the materno–fetal interface may be damped.[63]

Is the Uterus an Immunologically Privileged Site?

One interesting concept which might explain the immunological paradox of pregnancy is that the uterus could be "exempt" from the rules of transplantation immunity. Perhaps special anatomic features within or around the uterus inhibit the initiation or expression of immunological reactions. Locales with these characteristics are called "immunologically privileged sites."[64] The best known of these sites is the cheekpouch of the Syrian hamster, within which allografts are accepted. The best explanation for this phenomenon is that the pouch lacks lymphatics, and hence the afferent limb of the immune response is nonfunctional.

The anterior chamber of the eye is a privileged site in some (but not all) systems. Recent work in this area in the mouse has indicated that antigens placed in the anterior chamber not only do not lead to sensitization but instead lead to specific acquired tolerance,[65] at least in part via the development of suppressor cells. In addition, the cornea is often said to be an immunologically privileged site as corneally allografts are normally not rejected. Since, however, such grafts are destroyed if the transplant becomes vascularized, it is clear that the privileged nature of the graft and its bed exist by virtue of their being avascular.

In the situations described above, the general procedure is to place the graft into an unsensitized host. The failure of graft rejection might reflect the inability to develop either the afferent or the efferent (or both) limbs of the immune response. To test the efferent limb in such situations, one can see whether allografted tissue put into immunologically privileged sites will remain undamaged if the host has been presensitized to the transplantation antigens of the graft. The answer is "no"; such tissues are usually rejected, presumably through antibody-mediated mechanisms.

Whether the uterus is an immunologically privileged site can be answered with certainty only through experiments in animals. Such experiments clearly show that allografts of cells or tissues placed into the uterus of a hormonally-prepared ("pseudopregnant") rat are rejected as they would be if placed in other sites.[26] Furthermore, the graft rejection mechanism causes hyperplasia of the parauterine lymph nodes and results in antigen-specific systemic sensitization of the host.

On the face of it, these ingenious experiments appear to establish the fact that the uterus is *not* an immunologically privileged site. Closer inspection, however, raises some doubts about this conclusion. A tissue placed in an allogeneic uterus is not a close analog of a fetus that develops in a very special environment, i.e., the placenta. Nor is the exogenous supply of pregnancy hormones a surrogate for the unique hormonal environment produced by the mother as well as by the fetoplacental unit. One might ask instead what would be the fate of an allograft placed *within the placenta.*

Such experiments have been done in rabbits by Dodd et al.[66] Although first set allogeneic skin grafts were rejected in 7–8 days when placed onto the skin of pregnant hosts, similar grafts put into the decidua were not rejected by 14 days (the time limit permitted by the experimental design). Furthermore, there was significant lymphocytic infiltration in the rejected grafts in the skin but not in the skin grafts in the decidua. These experiments strongly suggest that the decidual environment in a naive host does not support sensitization by allografts and/or expression of allograft immunity. If, however, skin allografts were placed into the decidua of previously sensitized pregnant recipients, they were rejected in 8 days. These latter results do not distinguish between cell-mediated or antibody-driven rejection mechanisms, but they do indicate that the *expression* of allograft immunity can be manifest in the decidual tissue. It must be recognized, however, that placing a graft into the decidua, where there is disruption of the tissue matrix, is quite different from having a "graft" like the fetus develop slowly while the decidua is also growing and developing. Thus although the experiments of Dodd are interesting, they necessarily have artificial aspects. It may be difficult to answer precisely whether the *decidua* represents an immunologically privileged situation.

Taken together, the results discussed above indicate that: first, the uterus, in itself, is not an immunologically privileged site, but second, the decidual environment is one in which primary allograft immunity is poorly developed, if at all, but one in which preexisting systemic allograft immunity can be expressed.

Fetal Immunocompetence

It is clear that immunocompetence in the fetus develops during uterine life and does not reach maturity until after birth. This phenomenon is most obvious in rodents, where the newborn pup is indeed severely immunodeficient. The immunodeficiency of the newborn is less pronounced in humans, however. Burnet[67] believed (correctly, I think) that the immaturity of the fetal immune system promotes tolerance to self-antigens, but there is enough immunocompetence—at least late in fetal life to be important in terms of materno–fetal relations.

Fetal cellular responses can be detected in the first trimester. Fetal T cells will respond to PHA at 10–12 weeks, can respond in an MLR at 12–15 weeks, and can develop into CTLs by 16 weeks.[68] The latter indicates that the fetus can develop alloreactivity to foreign MHC antigens—a point that will become important later.

Active sensitization of the fetus occurs.[69] This may be seen in both the cellular and the humoral compartments of the immune system. The sensitized state could be achieved either by transfer of antigen from the mother with a subsequent T and/or B cell response (active immunity), or it could occur via passive transfer of sensitized maternal T and/or B cells (passive immunity). (The passive transfer of maternal immunoglobulin has been discussed in Chapter 2). If maternal T and/or B cells can remain viable in the fetus, a state of stable chimerism might result, with the fetus able to use the mother's immunologic machinery "adoptively." This means that antigens to which the mother had responded would be immunogenic in the fetus and newborn by virtue of the presence of maternal immune machinery.

It is not always easy to distinguish between the transfer of antigens vs the transfer of lymphoid cells. Certainly if the transferred antigen is a microbe, the infected fetus can mount an active immune response, usually seen as specific IgM antibody. Cellular responses are more problematic. Early experiments showed that both maternal and cord blood lymphocytes proliferated when exposed to antigens in vitro. This result was taken as evidence that it was maternal cells in the cord blood that responded, as it was believed that the fetus would not have been exposed to the antigens in the study.[70] This conclusion is open to question as the antigens used have strong superantigen activities and would therefore not require prior exposure. A better protocol examined cultures of newborn PBL from mothers who had or did not have infections with *E. coli*. Cells from offspring of infected mothers responded to *E. coli* antigen by going into mitosis, whereas cells from offspring of uninfected mothers did not. Thus the responding cells from the offspring of infected mothers appear to be "memory cells" that have recognized and responded to microbial antigens that had crossed the placenta previously.[71] However, one can also interpret the results to mean that the responding cells in the cord blood of offspring from infected mothers were in fact maternal *E. coli*-primed cells. Better conclusions can be drawn from those few newborns of tuberculin-positive mothers who were also tuberculin positive.[69] The fact that this sensitivity was short-lived strongly suggests that it was mediated by maternal T cells that did not survive to any degree after birth.

The implication of these data is important. It provides grounds for believing that foreign maternal cells will not ordinarily survive in the normal fetus late in pregnancy or in the puerperium. That is, the late fetus and newborn have the capacity to remove maternal cells, thus *not* providing the setting for a stable maternal chimera, or for possible GVHD. As mentioned above, the ability of fetal cells to respond in MLR cultures is a strong argument in favor of at least some degree of fetal alloreactivity.

Summary

A decrease in maternal immunocompetence during pregnancy has been suggested as a factor that contributes to the success of the fetal allograft.

1. The maternal immunologic response in pregnancy.
    a. Maternal immune responses to infection are, in most cases, adequate in pregnancy.
    b. Humoral and cell-mediated responses to conventional antigens are generally normal in pregnancy.
    c. The immunologic machinery, e.g., T and B cells and their products, are not significantly altered in pregnancy.
2. Immunoregulatory mechanisms in pregnancy.
    a. Pregnancy-associated hormones include steroid hormones, alpha-fetoprotein, and trophoblast-derived molecules.
    b. Many of these materials have immunosuppressive properties in vitro, but their in vivo relevance to fetal allograft survival is not clear.
    c. Suppressor cells and substances have been seen in the pregnancy plasma, PBL, decidua, and in cord blood. Their nature and influence on fetal survival is just beginning to be understood.
3. The uterus as an immunologically privileged site.
    a. Normal humoral and cellular immune responses can occur within the uterus itself, either in the pregnancy or nonpregnant state.
    b. The possibility that the decidual environment (distinct from the extra-decidual uterine environment) is immunologically privileged is still unsure.

References

1. Weinberg ED: Pregnancy: Associated depression of cell-mediated immunity. *Rev Infect Dis* 1984; 6: 814–831.
2. Brabin BJ: Epidermiology of infection in pregnancy. *Rev Infect Dis* 1985; 7: 579–603.
3. Drutz DJ, Catanzaro A: Coccidioidomycosis. *Am Rev Respir Dis* 1978; 117: 727–771.

4. Falkoff R: Maternal immunologic changes during pregnancy: A critical appraisal. *Clin Rev Allergy* 1987; 5: 287–300.
5. Stagno S, Reynolds DW, Huang E-S, et al: Congenital cytomegalovirus infection: Occurrence in an immune population. *N Engl J Med* 1977; 296: 1254–1258.
6. Hedvall E: Pregnancy and tuberculosis. *Acta Medica Scand* 1953; 147 (Suppl. 286): 3–101.
7. Murray DL, Imagawa DT, Okada DM, et al.: Antibody response to monovalent A/New Jersey/8/76 influenza vaccine in pregnant women. *J Clin Microbiol* 1979; 10: 184–187.
8. Amino N, Kuro R, Tanizawa O, et al: Changes of serum antithyroid antibodies during and after pregnancy in autoimmune thyroid diseases. *Clin Exp Immunol* 1978; 31: 30–37.
9. Exon PD, Dixon K, Malins JM: Insulin antibodies in diabetic pregnancy. *Lancet* 1974; i: 126–128.
10. Jones WR, Hawes CS, Kemp AS: Studies on cell-mediated immunity in human pregnancy, in Wegmann TG, Gill III TJ (eds): *Immunology of Reproduction.* New York, Oxford University Press; 1983: 363–381.
11. Lichtenstein MR: Tuberculin reaction in tuberculosis during pregnancy. *Am Rev Tuberc* 1942; 46: 89–92.
12. Strelkauskas AJ, Wilson BS, Dray S, et al: Inversion of human T and B cell levels in early pregnancy. *Nature* 1975; 258: 331–333.
13. Moore MP, Carter NP, Redman CW: Lymphocyte subsets in normal and pre-eclamptic pregnancies. *Br J Obstet Gynaecol* 1983; 90: 32–331.
14. Bardeguez AD, McNerney R, Frieri M, et al: Cellular immunity in preeclampsia: Alterations in T-lymphoycte subpopulations during early pregnancy. *Obstet Gynecol* 1991; 77: 859–862.
15. Coulam C, Silverfield J, Kazmar R, et al: T lymphocyte subsets during pregnancy and the menstrual cycle. *Am J Reprod Immunol* 1983; 4: 88–90.
16. Degenne D, Canepa S, Lecomte C, et al: Serial study of T-lymphocyte subsets in women during very early pregnancy. *Clin Immunol Immunopathol* 1988; 48: 18–191.
17. Lucivero G, Selvaggi A, Dell'osso S, et al: Mononuclear cell subpopulations during normal pregnancy. I. Analysis of cell surface markers using conventional techniques and monoclonal antibodies. *Am J Reprod Immunol* 1983; 4: 142–145.

18. Tallon DF, Corcoran DJD, O'Dwyer EM, et al: Circulating lymphocyte subpopulations in pregnancy: A longitudinal study. *J Immunol* 1984; 132: 1784–1787.

19. Feinberg BB, Gonik B: General precepts of the immunology of pregnancy. *Clin Obstet Gynecol* 1991; 34: 3–16.

20. Nelson JH, Lu T, Hall JE, et al: The effect of trophoblast on immune state of women. *Am J Obstet Gynecol* 1973; 117: 689–699.

21. Covelli HD, Wilson RT: Immunologic and medical considerations in tuberculin-sensitized pregnant patients. *Am J Obstet Gynecol* 1978; 132: 256–259.

22. Krause PJ, Ingardia CJ, Pontius LT, et al: Host defense during pregnancy: Neutrophil chemotaxis and adherence. *Am J Obstet Gynecol* 1987; 157: 274–280.

23. Vaquer S, de la Hera A, Jorda J, et al: Diminished natural killer activity in pregnancy: Modulation by interleukin 2 and interferon gamma. *Scand J Immunol* 1987; 26: 691–698.

24. Ogra PL, Ogra SS: Local antibody response to poliovirus in the human genital tract. *J Immunol* 1973; 110: 1307–1311.

25. Ogra PL, Yamanaka T, Losonsky GA: Local immunologic defenses in the genital tract, in Gleicher N (ed): *Reproductive Immunology.* New York, Alan R. Liss, Inc.; 1981: 381–394.

26. Beer AE, Billingham RE: Host responses to intra-uterine tissue, cellular and fetal allografts. *J Reprod Fertility* 1974; 21: 59–50.

27. Hetherington CM: The absence of any effefct of maternal/fetal incompatibility at the H-2 and H-3 loci on pregnancy in the mouse. *J Reprod Fertil* 1973; 33: 135–139.

28. Gottesman SRS, Stutman O: Comparison of cellular immune changes in the draining paraaortic lymph nodes in syngeneic and allogeneic pregnancies, in Gleicher N (ed): *Reproductive Immunology.* New York, Alan R. Liss, Inc.; 1981: 121–136.

29. Hench PS: The reversibility of certain rheumatic and non-rheumatic conditions by the use of cortisone or of the pituitary adrenocorticotrophic hormone. *Ann Int Med* 1952; 36: 1–38.

30. Claman HN: Corticosteroids and lymphoid cells. *N Engl J Med* 1972; 287: 388–397.

31. Claman HN: Glucocorticoids and autoimmune disorders, in Schleimer RP, Claman HN, Oronsky AL (eds): *Anti-inflammatory Steroid Action: Basic and Clinical Aspects.* San Diego, Academic; 1989: 409–422.

32. Klopper A: Pregnancy proteins and hormones in the immune response of pregnancy, in Stern CMM (ed): *Immunology of Pregnancy and its Disorders.* Dordrecht, Kluwer Academic Publishers; 1989: 91–113.
33. Gall SA: Maternal adjustments in the immune system in normal pregnancy. *Clin Obstet Gynecol* 1983; 26: 521–536.
34. Clemons LE, Siiteri PK, Stites DP: Mechanisms of immuno-suppression of progesterone on maternal lymphocyte activation during pregnancy. *J Immunol* 1979; 122: 1978–1985.
35. Murgita RA, Tomasi TB: Suppression of immune response by alpha-fetoprotein. *J Exp Med* 1975; 141: 440–449.
36. Wajner M, Pailha SS, Wagstaff TI: Inhibition of mitogen and allogeneic stimulated lymphocyte growth by human amniotic fluid: Lack of correlation between a-fetoprotein level and *in vitro* immunosuppression. *Eur J Obstet Gynecol Reprod Biol* 1986; 21: 225–232.
37. Menu E, Chaouat G: Immunoregulatory factors secreted by human or murine placenta or gestational tumors, in Chaouat G (ed): *The Immunology of the Fetus.* Boca Raton, FL, CRC Press, Inc.; 1990: 153–160.
38. Johannsen R, Haupt H, Bohn H, et al: Inhibition of the mixed leukocyte culture (MLC) by proteins: Mechanism and specificity of reaction. *Z Immuno Forsch Exp Therap* 1976; 152: 280–285.
39. Kasakura S: A factor in maternal plasma during pregnancy that suppresses the reactivity of mixed leukocyte cultures. *J Immunol* 1971; 107: 1296–1301.
40. Garcia DC, Moreno A, Palomino P: The effect of human pregnancy serum on the synthesis and action of interleukin-1. *J Reprod Immunol* 1988; 13: 17–30.
41. Nicholas NS, Panayi GS: Human pregnancy serum inhibits interleukin-2 production. *Clin Exp Immunol* 1984; 58: 587–595.
42. Smart YC, Roberts TK, Clancy RL,et al.: Early pregnancy factor: Its role in mammalian reproduction. *Fertil Steril* 1981; 35: 397–402.
43. Whyte A, Heap RP: Early pregnancy factor. *Nature* 1983; 304: 121–122.
44. Morton H, Rolfe BE, Cavanagh AC: Ovum factor and early pregnancy factor. *Recent Adv Mammal Develop* 1987; 23: 73–92.

45. Granberg C, Hirvonen T, Toivanen P: Cell-mediated lympholysis by human maternal and neonatal lymphocytes: Mother's reactivity against neonatal cells and vice versa. *J Immunol* 1979; 123: 2563–2567.

46. Genetet N, Genetet B, Amice V, et al: Allogeneic responses in vitro induced by fetomaternal alloimmunization. Am J *Reprod Immunol* 1982; 2: 90–96.

47. Vanderbeeken Y, Vlieghe MP, Duchateau J, et al: Suppressor T-lymphocytes in pregnancy. *Am J* Re*prod Immunol* 1984; 5: 20–24.

48. Kovithavongs T, Dossetor JB: Suppressor cells in human pregnancy. *Transplant Proc* 1978; 10: 911–913.

49. McMichael AJ, Sasazuki T: A suppressor T cell in the human mixed lymphocyte reaction. *J Exp Med* 1977; 146: 368–380.

50. Castilla JA, Vargas L, Garcia-Tortosa C, et al: Short-lived suppressor cell activity during normal human pregnancy. *J Reprod Immunol* 1990; 18: 139–145.

51. Wang H-S, Kanzaki H, Yoshida M, et al: Suppression of lymphocyte reactivity in vitro by supernatants of explants of human endometrium. *Am J Obstet Gynecol* 1987; 157: 956–963.

52. Lala PK, Kennedy TG, Parhar RS: Suppression of lymphocyte alloreactivity by early gestational human decidua. II. Characterization of the suppressor mechanisms. *Cell Immunol* 1988; 116: 411–422.

53. Lala PK, Kennedy TG, Parhar RS: Suppression of lymphocyte alloreactivity by early gestational decidua. I. Characterization of suppressor cells and suppressor molecules. *Cell Immunol* 1988; 116: 392–410.

54. Pace D, Morrison L, Bulmer JN: Proliferative activity in endometrial stromal granulocytes throughout menstrual cycle and early pregnancy. *J Clin Pathol* 1989; 42: 35–39.

55. Menu E, Kaplan L, Andreau G: Immunoactive products of human placenta. I. *Cell Immunol* 1989; 119: 341–352.

56. Segars JH, Niblack GD, Osteen KG, et al: The human blastocyst produced a soluble factor(s) that interferes with lymphocyte proliferation. *Fertil Steril* 1989; 52: 381–387.

57. Parhar RS, Yagel S, Lala PK: PGE2-mediated immuno-suppression by first trimester human dicidual cells blocks

activation of maternal leukocytes in the decidua with protential anti-trophoblast activity. *Cell Immunol* 1989; 120: 61–74.

58. Daya S, Clark DA: Production of immunosuppressor factor(s) by preimplantation human embryos. *Am J Reprod Immunol Microbiol* 1986; 11: 98–90.

59. Daya S, Johnson PM, Clark DA: Trophoblast induction of suppressor-type cell activity in human andometri tissue. *Am J Reprod Immunol* 1989; 19: 65–72.

60. Daya S, Clark DA, Devlin C, et al: Preliminary characterization of two types of suppressor cells in the human uterus. *Fertil Steril* 1985; 44: 778–785.

61. Daya S, Clark DA: Immunoregulation at the maternofetal interface: The role of suppressor cells in preventing fetal allograft rejection. *Immunol Allergy Clinics N Am* 1990; 10: 49–64.

62. Papadogiannakis N, Johnsen S-A, Olding LB: Suppressor cell activity in human cord blood, in Chaouat G (ed): *The Immunology of the Fetus.* Boca Raton, FL, CRC Press, Inc.; 1990: 216–227.

63. Billingham RE, Head JR: Recipient treatment to overcome the allograft reaction, with special reference to nature's own solution. *Prog Clin Biol Res* 1986; 224: 159–185.

64. Billingham RE, Silvers WK: *Immunobiology of Tissue Transplantation*, Englewood Cliffs, Prentice-Hall Inc.; 1971.

65. Niederkorn JY: Immune privilege and immune regulation in the eye. *Adv Immunol* 1990; 48: 191–226.

66. Dodd M, Andrew TA, Coles JS: Functional behavior of skin allografts transplanted to rabbit deciduomata. *J Anat* 1980; 130: 381–390.

67. Burnet M: *Cellular Immunology*, Melbourne, University Press; 1969: 213.

68. Lawton AR, Cooper MB: Ontogeny of Immunity, in Stiehm ER (ed): *Immunologic Disorders in Infants and Children.* Philadelphia, W. B. Saunders Co.; 1989: 1–14.

69. Cramer DV, Dunz M-W, Gill TG: Immunologic sensitization prior to birth. *Am J Obstet Gynecol* 1974; 120: 431.

70. Leikin S, Oppenheim JJ: Prenatal sensitization. *Lancet* 1971; 2: 876–877.

71. Brody JJ, Oski FA, Wallach EE: Neonatal lymphocyte reacting as an indicator of intrauterine bacterial contact. *Lancet* 1968; 1: 1396–1398.

Chapter 4

Maternal Immune Responses to Fetal Antigens

If there were a complete immunologic separation between mother and fetus, there would be no need for this chapter, because maternal immune responses to fetal antigens would not occur. The fact that they do occur indicates that the mother's immune system can respond to fetal antigens. However, the existence of such reactions does not tell us how they develop. They might originate locally, i.e., in or around the placenta, and then, because of the mobility of elements of the immune system (Chapter 1) result in a state of systemic sensitization. Or, they might originate from fetal-to-maternal cell traffic, in which case the sensitization would take place outside of the materno–fetal unit. Or, both mechanisms might operate.

In considering this subject, a number of variables are of interest. These variables include the frequency of maternal sensitization, the time at which it occurs, the relation to parity, and the intensity of sensitization. Other parameters of importance include the type of response (T or B cell), the nature of the stimulating antigens, the methods of demonstrating the sensitized state, and the possible existence of counter-sensitization pathways, such as tolerance or suppression. It should not be surprising that complete or even satisfying characterizations of these variables do not often exist.

Antibodies
to Fetal and Placental Antigens

By far the most work in this area has been done by looking at serum antibodies directed against fetal (paternal) antigens. This is because antibody-detection systems long preceded methods of measuring cellular responses, because serum is more easily obtained and stored than cells, and because the technology is simpler.

Leukoagglutinating Antibodies

Rose Payne[1] and Jon van Rood [2] and their colleagues were the first to demonstrate the presence of antipaternal antibodies in pregnancy sera. They both used the simple but sensitive *leukoagglutinin* method in which cells are suspended in maternal serum and cell clumping is the positive readout. Payne found leukoagglutinins in the sera of 18% of multiparas who had not received blood transfusions, and came to the conclusion that the antibodies resulted from fetal stimuli. van Rood also found leukoagglutinins in some multiparas. Women who had the antibodies had had an average of 7 pregnancies, whereas those who did not had an average of 3 pregnancies. These early studies raised many questions, but indicated right from the beginning that pregnancy is by no means always accompanied by the presence of alloantibodies. In fact, one could reasonably ask whether the "normal" pregnancy could be characterized by the presence of alloantibodies or by their absence.

Leukocytotoxic (Lymphocytotoxic) Antibodies

The leukoagglutination technique was soon superseded by the complement-dependent method that detected leukocytotoxic antibodies (LCAs). This refinement consists of mixing maternal serum and the appropriate target leukocytes (paternal or offspring), or third party and then adding a source of complement. The positive readout here is lysis of the target cells. This method is sensitive, rapid, and can be made quantitative. It is still the basic test used for HLA tissue typing. However, it will only be positive if the antibodies are IgM or IgG, as they are the only isotypes that fix complement. Although the test can measure cytolysis of many types of leukocytes, the target cells most often examined are lymphocytes. Thus, this is usually called lymphocytotoxic antibody assay.

Studies in the 1970s showed that 12% of primiparous women had LCAs when serum that had been taken at delivery was measured, and most LCAs appeared to be directed to paternal (rather than third party) antigens.[3] The specificity of LCAs from multiparas did not seem to differ from those of primiparas,[4] but the techniques for determining specificity were not far advanced. An important step was the realization that antipaternal antibodies could be eluted from the placenta,[5] giving rise to the concept of the "placental sink" for antiallotypic antibodies. This study also showed that serum alloantibody levels fell in the last trimester, suggesting that studies relying on sera taken at term[3] might give falsely low estimates of the incidence (or amount) of antipaternal antibodies.

When studies began to explore the effect of parity, it was found that the percentage of women with LCAs rose from 5% in the first pregnancy to a plateau of 15% after 3 or more pregnancies.[6] However, the serum samples were taken in the last trimester or a delivery, so that the placental sink phenomenon was undoubtedly a confounding factor. Another study, however, in which the sera were drawn before 20 weeks of gestation, gave similar results, with a peak LCA incidence of 24% during the third or later pregnancies.[7] In secundagravidae, antibodies occurred more often in women who had previously had a term pregnancy than in those who had previously had a spontaneous abortion. This indicates that the length of exposure to the fetus is important in determining the strength of the alloantibody response.[7]

LCAs were found to be mainly of the IgG isotype (and sometimes IgM) and they could be detected not only during pregnancy but also after skin graft rejection and blood transfusion.[8] Both agglutinating and cytotoxic tests might be positive.

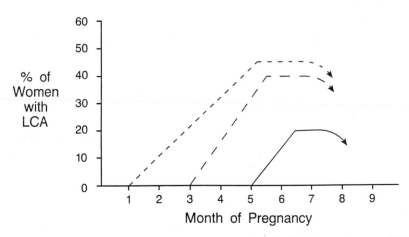

Fig. 1. LCA and pregnancy order. An idealized summary of the incidence of LCA by pregnancy. In the first pregnancy (solid line) LCA appears in the second trimester but are present in 20–25% of pregnancies. In second pregnancies (dashed line) and third pregnancies (dotted line) the incidence of LCA is higher and the antibodies appear earlier.

The increase in the incidence of LCAs with increasing parity has been confirmed[9] and is not surprising, as it appears to represent the results of "priming" by previous pregnancies.

More comprehensive studies traced the temporal development of LCAs. During the first pregnancy, no antibodies appeared until 5 months of gestation. The maximum incidence of LCAs was only 20% and this occurred at 6 months. Antibodies appeared earlier in the second pregnancy, i.e., at 3 months, but only 27% of mothers had them. In multiparas, there were no detectable antibodies at 1 month, 12% positivity at 2 months, and the maximum incidence of 33% was seen variably between 3–8 months. In all groups—primiparas, secondiparas, and multiparas—the frequency of LCA occurrence dipped in the last trimester.[10] Although the data in this paper present the frequency with which LCAs are found, and not the amount, the graphs can also be looked at as if the points represented titers of antibodies. An idealized representation of the findings is shown in Fig. 1.

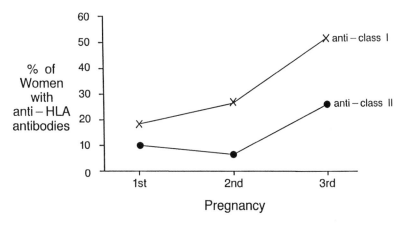

Fig. 2. Frequency of anti-HLA class I and class II antibodies by pregnancy order.

At least one study indicates that the incidence of LCAs may be higher, if one takes care to identify IgM antibodies. The activity of these antibodies are best identified at lower temperatures that many investigators did not use. By this method, no antibodies are seen in the first trimester of the first pregnancy, but they are eventually seen in 52% of primigravidas and in 76% of second and 85% of third pregnancies.[11] Nevertheless, although the presence of IgM LCAs may indicate maternal isosensitization, the antibodies will not cross the placenta, and so are of less interest than IgG antibodies. At any rate, although many multiparous women develop LCAs in their pregnancies, not all women do so. LCAs could not be seen in over half of the pregnancies.[12] This remained true when LCAs were differentiated into those directed against MHC class I antigens (HLA-A, B, and C) and those directed against class II (HLA-DR).[13] As shown in Fig. 2 the data from Morin-Papunen et al. indicate that antibodies against class I were more prevalent than those against class II. The frequency of both specificities rose from the first pregnancy onward, but never exceeded 50%. (It should be noted that the serum was taken at delivery.) It is not clear why no more than 50% of multiparas make LCAs. Leaving aside questions about the sensitivity of the methods, it is possible that some women are "nonresponders" in respect to making anti-HLA antibodies. Certain strains of mice fail to make anti-H-2 antibodies so the situation is not unique.[14] Another possibility, to be discussed below, is the blocking of anti-HLA antibodies by anti-anti-HLA antibodies, i.e., by anti-idiotypes.

Some work has been done to detect antibodies that merely bind paternal lymphocytes. This method obviates the requirement that the detected antibodies fix complement and thus lead to lysis of target cells. Such antibodies (not directed to HLA, however), were found in most primiparas (11/16 and all 11 multiparas tested).[15] This approach needs more attention, as it is likely that more sensitive and less exclusive testing methods may find that maternal antibodies are more prevalent than previously suspected.

MLR Blocking Antibodies

Another method of of determining anti-fetal or anti-paternal antibodies is to look at the effects of maternal serum on the mixed leukocyte reaction (MLR) Of 45 multiparas, 16 had serum that inhibited the MLR between mother and father.[16] In this and in another comparative study,[17] there were fewer sera with LCA activity than there were sera that inhibited the MLR. These data suggested that MLR inhibition is a more sensitive assay than LCA activity for detecting antipaternal antibodies.[18]

The kinetics of the development of MLR suppressive activity during pregnancy roughly parallels that of the development of LCA activity, but may rise more slowly. There was none from 9 to 20 weeks, more at 29 weeks, and still a greater incidence at 36 weeks.[19] In this study there did not seem to be a placental sink effect.

When a maternal serum is able to inhibit an MLR, the question arises as to which part of this complex reaction is being affected. Is the inhibitor blocking the stimulators or the responders? (A third possibility is that the target of inhibition might be a nonpolymorphic molecule, such as IL-2 or its receptor.) This question is of great importance in thinking about maternal–fetal interactions and their possible inhibition by maternal antibodies. If the "normal" (undesirable) situation represents a possible reaction of maternal T cells to paternally-derived fetal HLA antigens, then the blocking effect could be directed against either the fetal HLA or against the specific maternal T cells directed against those antigens. In the first case, maternal anti-fetal HLA might act to "blindfold" the HLA antigens so that they would not be recognized by maternal alloreactive T cells—a kind of immunological enhancement. In the second case, the antibodies would be directed against the TcR of those clones of maternal T cells that specifically react to the particular fetal HLA antigens. In this sense, the antibodies would act as anti-receptors, i.e., they would be anti-idiotypic, where the TcR serves as the idiotype. T cells with other alloreactive specificities mediated by different TcRs would be unaffected. A diagram of these possibilities is shown in Fig. 3.

Some studies have shown that MLR inhibition may be specific or nonspecific. One group found that MLR inhibition was most often directed at paternal rather than maternal stimulators, but inhibition of third party stimulators could also occur.[16] Another study gave a hint that inhibition of the responders might require higher concentrations of serum,[20] and that antistimulator activity might be more common than antiresponder activity. In another report,[17] out of the 50% percent of pregnancy sera that had any MLR blocking activity, there were more sera that blocked stimulators than blocked responders.

One group used the one-way MLR technique with IgG isolated from serum and from placental eluates. They tested the ability of these materials to block the MLR between cord blood stimulators and maternal responders, and asked whether the inhibitory properties were directed against T or B cells. Serum IgG blocked the MLR when B cells rather than T cells or unfractionated cells were stimulators. Placental eluate IgG inhibited the MLR regardless of whether the stimulators were T cell-enriched,

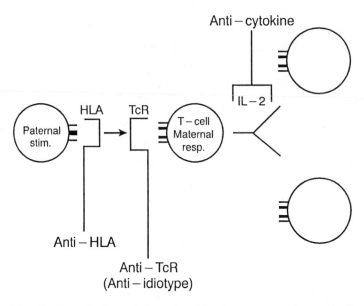

Fig. 3. Regulation of the mixed leukocyte reaction. Antibodies can inhibit the MLR at various points. In this schema, anti-HLA antibodies, antibodies to the TcR, and antibodies to cytokines such as IL-2 may each diminish the magnitude of the MLR.

B cell-enriched or unfractionated cord blood cells. They concluded that both individual and nonspecific blocking activities exist.[21] Similar conclusions were reached by another group,[22] and still another laboratory failed to find any specificity in placental eluates.[23]

Thus, maternal MLR blocking factors in serum or placental eluates appear to be directed mainly at paternal stimulators. Whether the factors are specific or nonspecific (or both) remains unsolved. Even if they turn out to be anti-HLA, what is the source of the antigens?

Anti-Idiotypic Antibodies and T Cells

Anti-idiotypic antibodies present a fascinating aspect of maternal–fetal alloreactivity. As mentioned above, the maternal B cell system has the capability (at least in principle) of producing antibodies not only to anti-HLA antibodies but also to the TcRs of those maternal T cell clones able to react to paternally-derived alloantigens on the fetus. These antibodies would then be able to block an MLR where cord blood leukocytes are the stimulators by blocking the responders; T cell reactions to unrelated alloantigens and to nonspecific mitogens or superantigens would be unaffected. These antibodies would be less effective in blocking MLRs where the stimulators are paternal cells rather than offspring cells. This is because the paternal cells would have stimulatory HLA antigens in both the inherited and the noninherited haplotype, yet there would not be expected to be anti-idiotpyes against the noninherited haplotype.

The subject of anti-idiotypic reactions in pregnancy has been explored in only a few laboratories because the experiments are technically difficult. In an extremely provocative and difficult paper, Suciu-Foca and colleagues [24] approached the question by asking whether the apparent absence of anti-HLA antibody (antibody-1) in so many pregnancies could be a result of the fact that anti-HLA reactivity is blocked by anti-anti-HLA (anti-idiotypes), i.e., antibody-2. They showed that serum from a postpartum woman that had anti-HLA antibodies had the anti-HLA reactivity blocked by sera harvested during another pregnancy. Presumably, this pregnancy serum had anti-anti-HLA from her (anti-idiotypic) antibody. The anti-anti-HLA activity developed as that pregnancy advanced, and appeared to "hide" the anti-HLA activity. They also showed that sera from parous women reacted against populations of activated T cells raised by stimulating mother's PBL with husband stimulators. These sera did not react against T cells activated by cells that were HLA-disparate from the husband. Thus the framework of the experiments was moved into the area of idiotypic and anti-idiotypic T cells. They showed that the putative anti-idiotypes in maternal serum blocked the autologous MLR that occurred when resting maternal T cells (the responders) were mixed with maternal cell populations enriched for T cells that had been primed by father stimulators. By analogy with the anti-idiotypic nomenclature originally devised for immunoglobulins, in this situation the father's HLA is the antigen, and the maternal T cells primed by the father's HLA is T cell-1, and its TcR is the idiotype. Finally, there is T cell-2, which responds specifically to the TcR on T cell-1 (which is specific for father's HLA) and thus T cell-2 is the anti-idiotypic *cell.* Thus, the experiment was designed to show that maternal PBL had responders that were anti-idiotypic T cell-2s, i.e., T cells against the anti-HLA TcR (idiotype) on the stimulators (T cell-1), which had been generated in turn in another culture by their interaction with paternal HLA. They interpreted their results as showing that pregnancy sera could have antibodies that blocked not only anti-HLA antibodies but also anti-HLA T cells.

Other results have been obtained in which pregnancy serum from a limited number of patients inhibited the MLR using father's stimulator cells. The results were interpreted as showing anti-idiotypic specificity but very large amounts of serum were required.[25] Other investigators reported results in which T cell clones reactive with father's cells were developed. IgG from the mother's pregnancy reacted with these T cell clones but not with control T cell clones alloreactive to other HLA antigens. Her serum blocked the MLR generated by father stimulator cells and her father-specific T cell clones but not her unrelated T cell clones. Finally, high concentrations of the Fab$_2$ fragment of her IgG bound to a father-specific T cell clone, blocked its cytolytic activity and stimulated that clone to proliferate.[26]

Taken together, these experiments suggest that maternal antipaternal antibody and T cell responses are common but are masked by anti-anti-paternal responses. They imply that the anti-idiotypic responses are beneficial because they block the possible harmful effects of antipaternal reactions. The above experiments were interpreted within the context of the HLA system, and a diagram of these concepts is shown in Fig. 4.

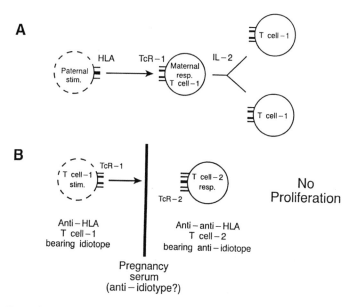

Fig. 4. Anti-idiotypic inhibition of the MLR. In the first MLR (A), maternal T cells complementary to paternal HLA are expanded (T cell-1). In B, these maternal T cell-1 are used as stimulators in a second MLR. If maternal T cells reciprocal to T cell-1, i.e., bearing anti-idiotype (i.e., T cell-2) are present, they will proliferate (not shown). However, if pregnancy serum containing anti-idiotypic antibodies are present, they will bind to T cell-1 and block the MLR.

Anti-TLX Antibodies

Anti-TLX antibodies have been described in Chapter 2. They are pertinent to this section on idiotypes because the current interpretation of this system involves idiotype regulation. Torry et al.[27] reported on a pregnancy serum that showed no antipaternal cytotoxic activity until after it had been adsorbed with material believed to contain anti-TLX antibody (which came, in turn, from a serum from a secondary aborter.) The adsorbed serum was now cytotoxic to husband's cells. The interpretation was that the pregnancy serum originally had both antibody-1 and antibody-2, but that adsorption with the secondary aborter anti-TLX (antibody-1) removed antibody-2 (anti-idiotype) leaving the patient's own antibody-1 (anti-TLX) to react with husband's cells, which contained the original antigen, TLX.

This work is extremely important in the understanding of alloreactivity in normal pregnancy. It suggests the presence of blocked anti-paternal reactivity. In this context, anti-TLX is inhibited by anti-idiotype, rather than by anti-HLA. A number of issues therefore are raised, in addition to those pertaining to the nature and polymorphism in the TLX system itself. It will be important to address the very same questions raised in the consideration of maternal-antipaternal HLA activity—the frequency, duration, intensity, immunoglobulin isotype, relation to parity, and so on, of these anti-idiotypic reactions.

Antibodies
to Trophoblast and Placental Antigens

Antibodies to trophoblast and placental antigens, other than TLX, have been detected. One laboratory found circulating antigen–antibody complexes in normal pregnancy and a lesser frequency of these in nulligravidae.[28] The antibodies, when dissociated from the complexes, reacted with syncytiotrophoblast cells. A sensitive enzyme-linked immunosorbent assay (ELISA) was developed, and it showed the presence of antibodies binding to trophoblast cells. As these antibodies were not adsorbed by PBL, they were presumably not of the HLA or TLX systems. Most of the antibody activity was in the form of immune complexes. In primiparas, the anti-trophoblast material was maximal in the first trimester, peaking at 5 weeks of gestation. After that, the IgM moiety disappeared, whereas the IgG isotype remained. The incidence of these antibodies lessened as parity increased.[29] Whether there is polymorphism in this antigen–antibody system, and what controls the incidence and level of the antibodies and immune complexes are unanswered questions. It is important to remember that the trophoblast has Fc receptors for IgG, so the binding of immunoglobulins to placental tissue does not necessarily mean that the antibodies in question have Fab fragments directed specifically to placental antigens.

Goto and colleagues[30] studied MLR-blocking sera from normal pregnancies and from habitually aborting women who had been immunized with allogeneic PBL. These sera blocked the MLR where the man was the stimulator and the woman was the responder. The blocking was removed by absorption with placental tissue, and autologous placenta was a better absorbant than allogeneic placenta. Yet, the absorption appeared to be unrelated to the HLA system (the TLX system was not mentioned). Assuming that it is the trophoblast tissue in the placenta that is absorbing the MLR blocking activity, these studies possibly suggest another candidate polymorphic system in the trophoblast that is not MHC.

Finally, one report, not yet confirmed, found noncytotoxic antibodies in pregnancy (and not in habitual aborters) that appear to block Fc receptors. Although not in themselves anti-HLA, family studies suggested that they are linked to HLA.[15]

Antibodies to Erythrocyte Antigens

Maternal *antibodies to erythrocyte antigens* on fetal cells represent another example of the mother's immune response to a polymorphic antigenic system. In theory, a woman not possessing one or more of a number of erythrocyte antigens that are present on the fetus could mount an immune response to any or all such antigens. In practice, however, there are a number of variables that determine whether the mother makes antibody (which is the only response usually measured), and if so, how much and what kind of antibody is made. Erythrocyte isoantigens differ in immunogenicity. The A and B antigens are the most immunogenic. Rh antigens are less potent but the consequences of Rh D isoimmunization are clinically more significant. Rh D is the most important antigen in the Rh family; the principles outlined here, however, also apply with respect to the less immunogenic molecules, Rh C and E. The next most immunogenic molecule is the Kell (K) antigen, which is one-tenth as immunogenic as Rh D.[31]

In the Rh system, maternal sensitization of Rh⁻ women occurs when fetal Rh⁺ bearing cells enter the maternal circulation. Data from studies in nonparous conditions show that small amounts of Rh D⁺ cells can induce detectable antibodies or can prime for antibody production in the future. As little as 0.1 mL of ABO compatible red cells will sensitize 3% of the recipients, and the incidence of sensitization rises with the dose of red cells.[32] Fetal red cells can enter the maternal circulation during the course of pregnancy so sensitization can occur in the first Rh-incompatible pregnancy. In first pregnancies of Rh⁻ women carrying ABO-compatible, Rh⁺ infants, about 8% developed detectable antibodies and another 9% were primed for subsequent antibody production.[33] One should clearly distinguish between the development of anti-Rh antibodies, which is not uncommon in the first pregnancy, and the incidence of clinical hemolytic disease of the newborn (HDN), which is uncommon. The greatest amount of erythrocyte transfer to the fetus occurs during transplancental hemorrhage at delivery, and the degree of immunization is enhanced by such things as toxemia, placental manipulation, or cesarian section. Nonetheless, all Rh⁻ people do not necessarily form anti-Rh antibodies, even if repeatedly exposed to Rh⁺ erythrocytes. These people can be considered to be "nonresponders" to this antigen, but the basis for this phenomenon is still unknown. The existence of nonresponders explains why, even though the incidence of Rh sensitization rises with increasing parity, there are some Rh⁻ women who never develop anti-Rh antibodies.

Rh⁺ erythrocytes are more immunogenic if the mother does not have antibodies to other antigens on the fetal cells, such as A or B. If she does, i.e., if there is ABO as well as Rh incompatibility, the A, B, or AB fetal red cells are opsonized with anti-A and/or anti-B and are quickly disposed of by the mother through nonimmunogenic pathways and therefore there is less opportunity for the immunodominant Rh molecules to sensitize. Thus, the dictum that "ABO incompatibility protects against Rh sensitization."

Isosensitization to A and B blood group antigens is more common than to Rh antigens. The isotypes of naturally-occurring anti-A and anti-B are curious. In A or B subjects, naturally occurring anti-B and anti-A (respectively) are mainly IgM, and would not cause fetal problems in any case. In group O subjects, however, the anti-A and anti-B may be mainly IgG (perhaps with some IgA antibody as well). The reasons for this difference in isotypes are obscure.[34] In 15% of Caucasian pregnancies, the mother is O-positive and the fetus has the A and/or B antigens. Thus, even in the first pregnancy, the incidence of ABO isosensitization and, to a lesser degree, of HDN is not negligible because all O-positive mothers have preexisting anti-A and anti-B. Because these antibodies are usually of the IgG isotype, they cross the placenta and can damage fetal cells. There are 2 features of pregnancy that tend to mitigate this undesirable situation. First, the placenta contains A and B antigens, which partially trap and neutralize maternal anti-A and anti-B. Second, the density of A and B antigens on fetal erythrocytes is low during embryonic life and does not reach adult levels until after birth.[34] Thus, these immature cells have fewer target molecules and would be less sensitive to antibody-mediated opsonization or lysis.

Isosensitization can develop to a large number of erythrocyte antigens other than those of the ABO and Rh families.[35] In general, the incidence both of such sensitization and of HDN is low, and HDN, when it occurs, tends to be mild. All of these features are a result of one or more of the following facts; the frequency of antigenic disparity between mother and fetus is low, the antigens are not immunologically potent, the antibodies produced are not IgG (reviewed in[35]). An exception to these generalizations is isosensitization to the Kell (K) antigen. K is not a frequently occurring antigen in the population. It can be responsible for the production of IgG antibodies that can cause severe HDN. However, it is paradoxical that the severity of HDN is not correlated with the anti-K titer.

The P antigens on erythrocytes comprise a complicated polymorphic system of glycolipids whose biochemistry is related to the ABO system. For our purposes, it is sufficient to note that most women have the phenotypes P_1 or P_2 and that these antigens are not known to cause fetomaternal problems. Rarely, however, a mother is of the p phenotype and makes "natural" anti-P_1PP^k antibodies. As the p phenotype is rare, it is almost certain that the fetus will contain P and/or P_1 antigens. If anti-P_1PP^k is of the IgG isotype, fetal damage may occur.[36,37]

T Cell Immune Responses
to Fetal and Placental Antigens

T cell responses are the major determinants of first and second set allograft rejection. Therefore, in terms of the survival of the fetus *as an allograft,* maternal T cell reactivity toward the fetus is a central problem. The question of whether there are maternal T cell responses that develop during pregnancy against fetal antigens is more difficult to deal with than the question of antibody responses to the fetus. This is because, at least for the major allelic system showing genetic polymorphism, i.e., MHC, the mother has T cell clones reactive to paternal HLA even before her first pregnancy. As mentioned in Chapter 1, T cell reactions to alloantigens probably represent crossreactions where the T cell clone was originally selected for its reactivity to self-HLA plus some nominal antigenic peptide. Therefore, right at the beginning of a pregnancy, a mother would have T cells able to recognize and respond to the paternal HLA haplotype expressed on the fetus. This form of "pre-existing" alloreactivity is not seen in the B cell system.

Cell-Mediated Immune Responses (CMI)

The expression of *cell-mediated immunity (CMI)* to allografts during pregnancy can no longer be measured in vivo in humans. Ideally, one would like to know the fate of a skin graft from a sibling placed on the mother when she is pregnant with another haploidentical sibling. From the results of animal experiments, we know that orthotopic skin grafts and even tissue grafts put into the uterus will be rejected. One might then ask whether the mother—as a consequence of the pregnancy—would have developed an increase in CMI to the fetal antigens. These experiments are difficult to do in this way, but the subject has been approached from a slightly different angle. Investigators determined the effect on a subsequent pregnancy of deliberately presensitizing the future mother to the fetal or maternal antigens. The methods used are ones that lead to accelerated graft rejection and the development of heightened MLRs and CTLs. Such presensitization experiments have been done in mice, rats, and rabbits and there was no effect: The subsequent pregnancies were normal. [38] Thus, even if one pregnancy did enhance the maternal CMI to fetal HLA antigens, there is no evidence that such a heightened alloreactive state would alter the course of the next pregnancy.

From the standpoint of fundamental T cell immunobiology, however, it is still of interest to pursue the question of whether the mother's alloreactivity is altered by the carriage of fetal alloantigens. In humans, this can best be done in vitro, looking at the MLR and at the development of CTLs. Thus, an in vitro T cell response can be analyzed into two phases: an early proliferative phase (the MLR) and a later effector response (the development of CTL).

Mixed Leukocyte Reactions (MLR)

If one serially studied the MLRs of mothers' T cells responding to fathers' stimulators during pregnancy, would there be an increase in reactivity and would it be specific? One study showed results in which the antipaternal MLR did increase as pregnancy advanced. As the response to third party stimulators did not change, this was interpreted as evidence for specificity. [39]

A different and rather original approach to this question asked whether there was increased MLR reactivity following pregnancy. Ten primiparous or multiparous women were studied postpartum together with their nulliparous sisters. These sisters were HLA-A, B, and C identical with the 10 index women. (DR typing was not done, but if siblings are HLA-A, B, and C identical, there as a very high probability that they will be DR identical as well.) The PBL of the index women and their siblings were used as responders in MLRs against stimulators from the respective fathers as well as from third parties. The question asked was whether the index women, as a result of their pregnancies, would have MLRs against their husbands' stimulating HLA that was different from their sisters' responses. There was no difference, indicating a lack of evidence that pregnancy caused any increase in HLA sensitization. (The MLRs were not done in pregnancy serum.)

A slightly different method of showing the results of possible allosensitization is to look for a *secondary (i.e. anamnestic) MLR* (Chapter 1), in parous women. So far, such reactions have not been found.[40,41]

Cytotoxic T Lymphocyte Responses (CTL)

Finally, one may ask if effector T cells with antipaternal cytolytic activity occur in pregnancy. Data are limited and the results are conflicting. A consensus of the experiments done so far is that antipaternal CTLs are uncommon and their presence does not prejudice the outcome of the pregnancy.[40,42]

Taken together, although these studies do not agree entirely, the bulk of the data fail to support the concept that pregnancy is accompanied by increased T cell reactivity to fetal antigens.

Suppressor Mechanisms, Cellular and Humoral

As mentioned in Chapter 1, antigen-specific and antigen-nonspecific suppressor influences are not difficult to demonstrate in immunological experiments, although the exact nature of the antigen-specific mechanisms is controversial. Thus, it is logical to look for suppressor activity in pregnancy. Chapter 3 has discussed various suppressor phenomena, namely *pregnancy serum* itself, and several *suppressor cells and factors* seen in the decidua and cord blood. One should add to this list the *anti-idiotypic antibodies* active against anti-HLA antibodies and TcRs and the antibody-2 in the *TLX* system.

The study of these suppressor phenomena is not well-advanced. One might consider that their presence is responsible for the lack of demonstrable maternal T cell activity to fetal antigens mentioned above, i.e., that suppressor mechanisms inhibit maternal alloreactivity. This concept, however, awaits proof. A more skeptical view is to consider that the suppressor mechanisms are mere epiphenomena. This concept is also unproven. To establish the irrelevance of suppressor mechanisms in pregnancy would entail making observations or manipulations that remove or overcome the suppressor mechanisms and then to show that the survival of the pregnancy had not been prejudiced.

Immunologic Tolerance in Pregnancy

Tolerance or unresponsiveness remains a central problem in immunology at present. Leaving aside systemic, nonspecific unresponsiveness (which is not present in pregnancy), can one see evidence for antigen-specific unresponsiveness? In nonpregnant conditions, mechanisms for this kind of tolerance include clonal deletion or anergy of T or B cells during ontogeny or after antigen or superantigen exposure, and suppressor T cells and downregulating B cell products, either anti-antigen or anti-idiotypic.

To a great extent, these topics have already been reviewed. There is no evidence that pregnancy involves a selective loss of T or B cell clones reactive to the fetus. But it is apparent that there are a variety of mechanisms already mentioned that tend to downregulate the antifetal responses. Whether this is called tolerance is really a semantic matter. In any event, the negative regulation of antifetal immunity is maximal at the local level, i.e., in the placenta, not systemically.

One can ask whether there is *any* kind of immunologic tolerance between mother and offspring. Before current regulations concerning human experimentation were in force, some data were obtained on the behavior of maternal, paternal, and child skin grafts. The available information shows that the mother's skin graft lasted longer on the child than did the father's skin, although both were eventually rejected.[43] This suggests that the child is somewhat tolerant of maternal transplantation antigens—a situation that might have occurred via transplancental passage of maternal HLA antigens. Conversely, however, the child's skin grafts placed on the mother lasted longer than expected, a result that was difficult to explain. This paper is frequently quoted but it is necessary to say that the data are difficult to interpret quantitatively. Besides, there could have been no HLA typing done in 1958, so the genetic relations between graft donor and recipient are not known. Still, this kind of experiment cannot be done today.

Mechanisms for Maternal Sensitization

Classical Immunological Sensitization Pathways

The material presented in the first part of this chapter shows that maternal sensitization to fetal alloantigens occurs frequently, as shown by the occurrence of anti-HLA antibodies. The mechanisms through which this takes place need discussion. Paternal (allogeneic) MHC antigens can be presented directly to MHC-specific responding maternal T cells. As the allogeneic class I or class II HLA molecules resemble "self-HLA plus X" (a nominal peptide), it seems that allogeneic MHC does not require the kind of antigen processing needed, for example, for protein antigens. Thus paternal HLA can be "presented" by the trophoblast cells themselves—class I being displayed to responding CD8$^+$ maternal cells and class II being displayed to CD4$^+$ cells, *if the MHC and the T cells have a chance to meet.*

The placental villous interstitium contains APCs capable of presenting paternally-derived alloantigen. If, however, there is a complete covering of the trophoblast by a layer of syncytiotrophoblast devoid of polymorphic HLA, the interstitial HLA-bearing APCs will remain sequestered from the maternal immune machinery. Thus, there may be no chance for the allogeneic HLA to meet the maternal T cells. This has been called *"immunological quarantine."*

How, then, is maternal sensitization accomplished? One possibility is via trophoblast deportation, after which HLA-bearing interstitial trophoblast cells have access to the peripheral immune system of the mother (*see* Chapter 2). However, although some parameters of trophoblast deportation are known, it is not clear whether these placental emboli actually cause maternal sensitization.

Another possibility is that HLA-bearing fetal peripheral blood leukocytes traverse the placenta, enter the maternal circulation and cause sensitization. Although the passage of fetal cells into the maternal blood occurs (*see* Chapter 2), neither the efficacy nor the efficiency of the immunization that occurs in this manner is known.

Still another point deserves comment. As allosensitization is facilitated by upregulation of class I and II expression, conditions favoring such upregulation may be accompanied by heightened degrees of alloreactivity. The development of placental "villitis," where inflammatory reactions undoubtedly cause increased cytokine production, may represent such a situation. "Villitis," although not a well-characterized entity, has been seen not only in "normal" pregnancies but more so in pre-eclampsia, intrauterine growth retardation, autoimmune states, and recurrent spontaneous abortion.[44] This subject needs more attention.

Nonclassical (Paraimmune?)
Maternofetal Interactions

The explosion of immunological knowledge has not only unraveled the roles of antigen-specific cells and molecules, but has also pointed out that there are potent antigen-nonspecific forces at work. Cytokines can be made and released by specific as well as nonspecific stimuli. NK cells can act without a classical CD3-associated TcR. These mechanisms may operate at the maternofetal interface even when antigen-specific molecules cannot be shown to play a role. Clark[45] has called this "paraimmunology." Whether indeed these mechanisms contribute to maternofetal recognition is a hypothesis worthy of study.

It is important to note that there is a dichotomy in the types of anti-paternal sensitization that occur in the mother. The absence of increased T-cell-mediated reactivity against the fetus is curious when compared to the frequent development of antibodies to paternal antigens carried on the fetus *(see above)*. A quick explanation for the disparity is not obvious. If trophoblast deportation causes the mother to make anti-paternal antibodies, why does it not cause the production of anti-paternal T cells? Or are they produced but masked in some way or hidden in anti-idiotypic reactions? The situation appears paradoxical and the solution to the paradox may well be instructive.

Summary

Pregnant women make a variety of immune responses to fetal antigens.
1. Antibodies can be made to fetal HLA antigens, to trophoblast and placental antigens, to erythrocyte antigens, and to putative TLX antigens.
   a. Not all pregnancies are associated with anti-fetal antibodies, and the variables determining the incidence and magnitude of these responses are not clear.

b. Anti-idiotypic antibodies have been described in a few instances. These may be directed to receptors for polymorphic antigens and may be important in fetal allograft survival.
2. T cell immune responses to fetal and placental antigens occur.
   a. Alloreactivity is present in the nonpregnant state.
   b. Increased T cell-mediated immunity toward the fetus does not occur in pregnancy.
3. Mechanisms for sensitizing the mother against fetal antigens include:
   a. Trophoblast deportation and leukocyte traffic across the placenta.
   b. Disruption of trophoblast sequestration in the decidua.

References

1. Payne R, Rolfs MR: Fetomaternal leukocyte incompatibility. *J Clin Invest* 1956; 37: 1756–1763.
2. van Rood JJ, Eernisse JG, van Leeuwen A: Leucocyte antibodies in sera from pregnant women. *Nature* 1958; 181: 1735–1736.
3. Tongio MM, Berrebi A, Pfeiffer B, et al.: Serological studies on lymphocytotoxic antibodies in primiparous women. *Tissue Antigens* 1971; I: 243–257.
4. Tongio MM, Berrebi A, Mayer S: A study of lymphocytotoxic antibodies in multiparous women having had at least four pregnancies. *Tissue Antigens* 1972; 2: 378–388.
5. Doughty RW, Gelsthorpe K: An initial investigation of lymphocyte antibody activity through pregnancy and in eluates prepared from placental material. *Tissue Antigens* 1972; 4: 291–298.
6. Ahrons S: HL-A antibodies: Influence on the human foetus. *Tissue Antigens* 1971; I: 121–128.
7. Burke J, Johansen K: The formation of HL-A antibodies in pregnancy: The antigenicity of aborted and term fetuses. *J Obstet Gynaecol Br Comm* 1974; 81: 222–228.
8. Ahrons S, Glavind-Kristensen S: Cytotoxic HL-A antibodies: Immunoglobulin classification. *Tissue Antigens* 1971; I: 129–136.

9.   Doughty RW, Gelsthorpe K: Some parameters of lymphocyte antibody activity through pregnancy and further eluates of placental material. *Tissue Antigens* 1976; 8: 43–48.

10. Vives J, Gelabert A, Castillo R: HLA antibodies and period of gestation: Decline in frequency of positive sera during last trimester. *Tissue Antigens* 1976; 7: 209–212.

11. Koening UD, Muller N: Occurrence and characterization of different types of cytotoxic antibodies in pregnant women in relation to parity and gestational age. *Am J Obstet Gynecol* 1983; 147: 671–675.

12. Regan L, Braude PR, Hill DP: A prospective study of the incidence, time of appearance and significance of anti-paternal lymphocytotoxic antibodies in human pregnancy. *Hum Reprod* 1991; 6: 294–298.

13. Morin-Papunen L, Tiilikainen A, Hartikainen-Sorri AL: Maternal HLA immunization during pregnancy: Presence of anti HLA antibodies in half of multigravidous women. *Med Biol* 1984; 62: 323–325.

14. Bell SC, Billington WD: Anti-fetal allo-antibody in the pregnant female. *Immunol Rev* 1983; 75: 5–30.

15. Power DA, Catto GRD, Mason RJ, et al: The fetus as allograft: Evidence for protective antibodies to HLA-linked paternal antigens. *Lancet* 1983; 2: 701–704.

16. Robert M, Betuel H, Revillard JP: Inhibition of the mixed lymphocyte reaction by sera from multipara. *Tissue Antigens* 1973; 3: 39–56.

17. Jonker M, van Leeuwen A, van Rood JJ: Inhibition of the mixed leukocyte reaction by alloantisera in man. II. Incidence and characteristics of MLC-inhibitory antisera from multiparous women. *Tissue Antigens* 1977; 9: 246–258.

18. Neppert J, Mueller-Eckhardt G, Neumeyer H, et al: Pregnancy-maintaining antibodies: Worshop report (Giessen, 1988). *J Reprod Immunol* 1989; 15: 159–167.

19. Bissenden JG, Ling NR, MacKintosh P: Suppression of mixed lymphocyte reactions by pregnancy serum. *Clin Exp Immunol* 1980; 39: 195–202.

20. Brochier J, Roitt IM, Festenstein H: Inhibition of lymphocyte proliferative responses by anti-HLA alloantisera. *Eur J Immunol* 1974; 4: 709–714.

21. Kajino T, Kanazawa K, Takeuchi S: Blocking effects of maternal serum-IgG and placental eluate-IgG on materno-fetal mixed lymphocyte reaction and their individual specificity. *Am J Reprod Immunol* 1983; 4: 27–32.

22. Hanaoka J-I, Takeuchi S: Individual specificity of blocking antibodies in molar and normal term placenta-bound IgG. *Am J Reprod Immunol* 1986; 3: 119–123.

23. Jeannet M, Werner C, Ramirez E, et al: Anti-HLA, anti-human "Ia-like" and MLC blocking activity of human placental IgG. *Transplant Proc* 1977; IX: 1417–1422.

24. Suciu-Foca N, Reed E, Rohowsky C, et al: Anti-idiotypic antibodies to anti-HLA receptors induced by pregnancy. *Proc Natl Acad Sci USA* 1983; 80: 830–834.

25. Singal DP, Butler L, Liao S-K, et al.: The fetus as an allograft: Evidence for antiidiotypic antibodies induced by pregnancy. *Am J Reprod Immunol* 1984; 6: 145–151.

26. Bonagura VR, Ma A, McDowell J, et al.: Anti-clonotypic autoantibodies in pregnancy. Cell Immunol 1987; 108: 356–365.

27. Torry DS, Faulk WP, McIntyre JA: Regulation of immunity to extraembryonic antigens in human pregnancy. *Am J Reprod Immunol* 1989; 21: 76–81.

28. Davies M: Antigenic analysis of immune complexes formed in normal human pregnancy. *Clin Exp Immunol* 1985; 61: 406–415.

29. Billington WD, Davies M: Maternal antibody to syncytiotrophoblast during pregnancy, in Wegmann TG, Gill III TJ (eds.): *Immunoregulation and Fetal Survival.* New York, Oxford University Press; 1987: 15–26.

30. Goto S, Takakuwa K, Kanazawa K, et al: MLR-blocking antibodies are directed against alloantigens expressed on syncytiotrophoblasts. *Am J Reprod Immunol* 1989; 21: 50–53.

31. Kevy SV: Rh hemolytic disease of the newborn, in Bern MM, Frigoletto FDJ (eds.): *Hematologic Disorders in Maternal Fetal Medicine.* New York, NY, Wiley-Liss; 1990:129–151.

32. Bowman JM: Alloimmune hemolytic disease of the newborn, in Williams WJ, Beutler E, Erslev AJ, Lichtman MA (eds.): *Hematology.* New York, McGraw-Hill; 1990: 687–693.

33. Bowman JM, Chown B, Lewis M, et al.: Rh isoimmunization during pregnancy: Antenatal prophylaxis. *Can Med Assn J* 1978; 118: 623–627.
34. Mollison PL, Engelfriet CP, Contreras M: *Blood Transfusion in Clinical Medicine*, Oxford, Blackwell Scientific; 1987: 315.
35. Konugres AA: Non-Rh hemolytic disease of the newborn, in Bern MM, Frigoletto FDJ (eds.): *Hematologic Disorders in Maternal Fetal Medicine*. New York, NY, Wiley-Liss; 1990: 153–169.
36. Marcus DM, Kundu SK, Suzuki A: The P blood group system: Recent progress in immunochemistry and genetics. *Semin Hematol* 1981; 18: 63–71.
37. Race RR, Sanger R: *Blood Groups in Man*, Oxford, Blackwell Scientific Publishing Co.; 1975: 139.
38. Billingham RE: Transplantation immunity and the maternal-fetal relation. *N Engl J Med* 1964; 270: 667–672.
39. Birkeland SA, Kristoffersen K: The fetus as an allograft: A longitudinal study of normal human pregnancies studied with mixed lymphocyte cultures between mother-father and mother-child. *Scand J Immunol* 1980; 11: 311–319.
40. Redman CWG, Arenas J, Mason DY, et al.: Maternal alloimmune recognition of the fetus in human pregnancy, in Wegmann TG, Gill III TJ (eds.): *Immunoregulation and Fetal Survival*. New York, Oxford University Press; 1987: 210–229.
41. Moore MP, Sargent IL, Ting A, et al.: Maternal cell-mediated immunity in pregnancy: Lymphocyte responses of mothers and their non-pregnant HLA-identical sisters to paternal HLA. *Clin Exp Immunol* 1983; 54: 91–94.
42. Sargent IL, Redman CWG: Maternal immune responses to the fetus in human pregnancy, in Stern CMM (ed.): *Immunology of Pregnancy and Its Disorders*. Dordrecht-Boston-London, Kluwer Academic Publishers; 1989: 115–141.
43. Peer LA: Behavior of skin grafts exchanged between parents and offspring. *Ann N Y Acad Sci* 1958; 73: 584–589.
44. Labarrere CA: Allogeneic recognition and rejection reactions in the placenta. *Am J Reprod Immunol* 1989; 21: 94–99.
45. Clark DA: Paraimmunology in the decidua? *Am J Reprod Immunol* 1990; 24: 37–39.

Chapter 5

Maternal Immune Responses Affecting Pregnancy and the Fetus

In thinking about the immunology of human pregnancy, it is of considerable interest to consider a variety of immunological changes, situations, and disorders in which the immune system of the mother affects the fetus. These situations are quite different from the question of materno–fetal allorecognition. They present us with insights into the pathogenesis of various conditions because of the unique nature of materno–fetal interactions. This chapter will include immune syndromes peculiar to pregnancy, such as hemolytic disease of the newborn (HDN) and related isoimmune syndromes, the effect of autoimmune diseases on pregnancy and on the fetus, as well as the effect of pregnancy on the autoimmune processes. It will touch on some miscellaneous topics, such as graft-vs-host disease and pre-eclampsia, which is considered by some to have an immune pathogenesis.

Hemolytic Disease of the Newborn and Related States

The basic nature of maternal sensitization to polymorphic erythrocyte allelic products has been discussed in Chapter 4. It should be mentioned, particularly in regard to the Rh system, that maternal isosensitization to Rh antigens proves that fetal cells gain access to the maternal immune system, that such antigens are recognized and that a measurable immune response, often with profound immunopathogenic consequences, often ensues. As human erythrocytes do not carry MHC antigens (unlike the situation in the mouse), the existence and mechanisms of Rh sensitization do not really provide direct help in understanding HLA isosensitization.

Rh Isosensitization

From an immunologist's point of view, the history of the development of our knowledge of Rh immunity represents a rarely-equaled success story. This story begins in the 1930s with the realization that hydrops fetalis, severe neonatal jaundice and kernicterus, and neonatal hemolytic anemia were all manifestations of a single disease, named erythroblastosis fetalis. In the 1940s, some astute observations and powerful reasoning by Levine and colleagues led to the conclusion that erythroblastosis was caused by maternal isosensitization by fetal Rh antigens.[1] In the 1950s, exchange and later intrauterine transfusions became accepted treatments for HDN and in the 1960s, the introduction of anti-Rh D immune globulin (RhIg) provided effective prophylaxis. This remarkable record indicates that in a span of 40 years, a disease was identified, its etiology and pathogenesis were elucidated, treatment was devised and, finally, a means of prevention was developed. Ideally, HDN caused by Rh isosensitization (HDN-Rh) should no longer exist, and indeed, it is now very uncommon. The medical profession as a whole (and not just pediatricians, hematologists, and immunologists) should be proud of this achievement.

Most cases of HDN-Rh are a result of the development of IgG antibodies to fetally-derived RhD^+ erythrocytes in a mother who is RhD^-. These antibodies cross the placenta and cause hemolysis and sometimes kernicterus and hydrops fetalis. The risk of Rh immunization depends on the amount of fetal blood entering the maternal circulation during pregnancy or at delivery. It also depends on the ABO status of the mother and child; ABO incompatibility "protects" against HDN-Rh, as a mother with natural IgM antibodies to A and/or B substances will rapidly clear fetal red cells bearing these antigens regardless of their Rh content.

Treatment with exchange transfusions is designed to "wash out" the IgG-coated fetal cells and the maternal IgG from the newborn circulation. Prophylactic treatment of RhD-women with RhIg after carriage of an RhD$^+$ pregnancy is designed to opsonize and remove any circulating fetal erythrocytes so that they do not reach the mother's immune system.

ABO and Other
Erythrocyte Isosensitization Syndromes

Much of what has been learned about these situations has come by analogy from studies in Rh incompatibility. ABO isosensitization is in fact the most common kind of erythrocyte incompatibility because of the frequency of pregnancies in which the fetus has an ABO antigen that the mother lacks, and because group O women lacking A or B substances have antibodies to them. Isosensitization to red cell antigens other than Rh and ABO are also briefly discussed in Chapter 4, and antibodies in the P system are discussed in Chapter 6.

Since the naturally-occurring anti-A and anti-B antibodies possessed by group O women are IgM, they will destroy immigrant fetal red cells containing A or B substances, but these antibodies will not cross the placenta to the fetus. Should the mother develop IgG antibodies against A or B substances, these would be capable of entering the fetal circulation and causing hemolytic anemia.

Antiglobulin Tests

The development of antiglobulin tests by Coombs greatly helped not only our understanding of the pathogenesis of isosensitization states but their management as well. These so-called "Coombs tests" are separated into direct antiglobulin tests

(DAT) and indirect antiglobulin tests (IAT). The DAT detects the presence of immunoglobulin on red cells. Since erythrocytes do not have FcRs, a positive DAT indicates that antibodies to some component of the red cell surface are binding by way of their Fab segments. The antigens can be intrinsic to the red cell (e.g., A, B, or Rh) or adsorbed onto that surface (e.g., C3 fragments generated during a complement-activating antigen-antibody reaction). The IAT detects antibodies in the serum that will adsorb onto red cells bearing the appropriate antigen. Obviously, a person with anti-erythrocyte antibodies in the serum who has red cells carrying those antigens may have both a positive DAT and IAT. This occurs in the fetus with HDN. Conversely, an Rh- pregnant woman, sensitized by her Rh$^+$ fetus will have only a positive IAT since her anti-Rh antibodies will not bind to her own Rh$^-$ red cells. By the careful choice of reagents, Coombs tests can be manipulated so that the immunohematologist can determine the isotype of the immunoglobulin responsible for the positive test results as well as the antigen to which it is directed.

Coombs tests teach some lessons to the pregnancy immunologist. A positive DAT indicates only that there are immunoglobulins on the erythrocytes, i.e., that they are opsonized. A positive DAT *suggests* that the life span of such opsonized red cells may be shorter than normal but it does not prove that point and it certainly does not make a diagnosis of HDN.

In Rh isosensitization, there is a general correlation between the degree of positivity of the Coombs tests and the presence and severity of HDN. In ABO incompatibility, however, the Coombs serological results are not predictive of HDN or even of hemolysis. Infants with ABO HDN can have only weak DATs. This may be partly because the antibody has only low affinity for the A and B antigens or because the number of such antigens on the newborn red cells is low. Both of these situations might lead to a loss of the antibodies from the red cell surface during the cell washing, which occurs in performing the DAT. Conversely, a positive cord blood DAT does not necessarily indicate HDN.

The incidence of positive cord blood DATs is 5% but the incidence of ABO HDN is only 0.7%.[2]

This may therefore be the place to emphasize that a positive immunological result in vitro, whether it be the presence of anti-erythrocyte antibodies, or anti-HLA antibodies, or anti-idiotypic antibodies, or inhibition of an MLR does not necessarily imply that the positive test has important in vivo consequences. That has to be established separately.

Neonatal Alloimmune
or Isoimmune Thrombocytopenic Purpura (NAITP)

This term denotes a situation in which the mother develops antibodies to foreign antigens on fetal platelets. It is not common, but when present, there is the possibility of intracranial hemorrhage in the newborn because of trauma to the head during vaginal delivery. These syndromes occur because of alloimmunization during pregnancy and should be differentiated from *autoimmune* (often called *idiopathic*) *thrombocytopenic purpura* (AITP), which is a primarily disease in the mother, unrelated to pregnancy in its pathogenesis, but of course able to complicate pregnancy *(see below)*.

NAITP occurs because of antigenic polymorphic systems involving platelets. Platelets contain three sets of antigens, although more may be discovered in the future. Rh antigens occur on platelets but erythrocyte-borne Rh antigens are more important. MHC class I molecules, namely HLA A and B, are found on platelet membranes, but HLA DR is not. Platelet-associated HLA alloantigens are highly immunogenic. This is reflected by the relative ease with which antiplatelet antibodies can be generated when random platelet transfusions are given, for instance during the thrombocytopenia of cancer chemotherapy. However, clinical alloimmune thrombocytopenic purpura in pregnancy is rarely caused by anti-HLA antibodies. Although 77 of 556 women had antiplatelet antibodies that were directed to HLA antigens, the only one of the babies who had purpura had antibodies to a platelet-specific antigen (although platelet counts were not routinely done on the infants).[3] As discussed earlier, the failure of maternal anti-HLA antibodies to affect the fetus is probably owing to the absorption of anti-HLA antibodies by the respective antigens in the placenta.

Platelet-specific antigens include PLA-1 and -2, PLE-1, and -2, DUZ0, KO[a], KO[b], and Bak[a] and Lek[a4]. Of these, PLA-1 is the most immunogenic, and it accounts for 50–80% of cases of NAITP. Although 1.3–3% of mothers are PLA-1[-], isoimmune thrombocytopenic purpura to this antigen nevertheless is still quite uncommon.[5,6] When maternal IgG antibodies to fetal platelets enter the fetal or perinatal circulation, fetal platelets are opsonized and removed by the reticuloendothelial system. The severity of the NAITP will depend on the amount and isotype of the antibody, the antigenic density on the platelet, the efficiency of the baby's reticuloendothelial system, and the compensatory power of the baby's bone marrow. The thrombocytopenia often appears in the first pregnancy and may be severe.[6] An unusual case of severe combined immunodeficiency (SCID) and GVHD was attributed to maternal anti-platelet antibodies suppressing the fetal immune system[7] *(see below)*.

Pemphigoid Gestationis

Pemphigoid gestationis (PG) was previously called herpes gestationis. There is no evidence that it has a herpetic or even a viral etiology, so the older term should be dropped. It is a rare polymorphic pruritic eruption that usually appears in the second trimester or later, but occasionally occurs earlier or even postpartum. Histologically, there is a mixed inflammatory infiltrate and immunohistochemical staining shows the presence of IgG and complement components at the dermo-epidermal junction. The IgG autoantibodies can be found in the circulation and they localize in the skin in a pattern similar to that seen in bullous pemphigoid.[8] The autoantibody is found in cord blood and there are some cases of neonatal pemphigoid gestationis.[9] The etiology of this syndrome is unclear. It occurs in the context of other autoimmune diseases as well as in hydatidiform mole and choriocarcinoma. The latter conjunctions suggest that it is a maternal response to trophoblastic antigens. Whether PG shows an increased association with HLA B-8, DR-3, or DR-4 and whether there is excessive fetal wastage is disputed.[10,11]

Organ-Specific Maternal Autoimmunity

There are a number of autoimmune syndromes where the specificity of the antibodies dictates that certain organs will be affected, at least primarily. It would be expected that the effects of pregnancy and the disease on each other will be somewhat different than in the systemic autoimmune diseases.

Autoimmune Thrombocytopenic Purpura (AITP)

This syndrome was usually called idiopathic thrombocytopenic purpura (ITP) in the older literature. As the techniques for demonstrating anti-platelet antibodies have improved, it has been recognized that these are antibody-mediated conditions. They are to be distinguished from neonatal alloimmune thrombocytopenia (discussed above) and from immune thrombocytopenias associated with drug allergy or platelet transfusions. The exact mechanisms that lead to autosensitization are unknown. The condition may arise within the context of another autoimmune syndrome, e.g., SLE, in which case the variables are usually those of SLE itself. Often, however, it occurs in seeming isolation. The general setting in pregnancy is one in which a woman who already has AITP, treated or not, becomes pregnant. The specificity of her anti-platelet antibodies is broad and not polymorphic, i.e., no anti-HLA or anti-PLA-1 antibodies are detected.[12] Therefore, if the antibodies are IgG (and they usually are), they will cross the placenta and affect the fetus and newborn as they affect the mother. The newborn may become thrombocytopenic. In general, the newborn's platelet count correlates best with the mother's titer of serum anti-platelet antibodies and neither with her platelet-associated antibody nor with her own platelet count. Thus the paradoxical situation can exist where the mother has a normal platelet count but the baby has thrombocytopenia.[12] A review of 122 pregnancies in AITP indicated that the danger to the mother was minimal, there having been no maternal deaths since 1951, when corticosteroids was first used to treat this problem. The fetal mortality, however, was 18%, with deaths owing to stillbirth, spontaneous abortion, and fetal hemorrhage.[13]

Autoimmune Hemolytic Anemia (AIHA)

As with AITP, autoimmune hemolytic anemia can occur as part of another autoimmune syndrome (again, with SLE) or as an isolated disease. When it occurs, for instance, as part of SLE, the pathogenesis is that of the transfer of IgG anti-erythrocyte antibodies to the fetus, with subsequent sequestration and hemolysis. AIHA arising *de nova* in pregnancy in the absence of a generalized autoimmune syndrome is very uncommon. Although there is disagreement on this point, the largest study indicates that it is often mild and may not require active treatment.[14]

Myasthenia Gravis

Myasthenis gravis (MG) is an autoimmune syndrome where muscular weakness is caused by antibodies affecting the acetylcholine receptors (AChR) at the neuromuscular junction. Because of these antibodies, neuromuscular transmission is blocked and the receptors themselves may be damaged or destroyed, by complement dependent or independent mechanisms.[15] Although it is difficult to correlate the severity of disease in different patients by comparing their titers of anti-AChR antibodies, the waxing and waning of muscular weakness in a given patient does correlate with changes in autoantibody titers. Interestingly, it is the occurrence of neonatal myasthenia gravis, caused by maternal antibodies, which gives the best indication that the antibody is probably the only autoimmune effector in the disease. This concept contrasts with some other autoimmune diseases, such as SLE and thyroiditis, where it is not clear how many of the anti-self processes are cellular and how many are humoral.

Myasthenia gravis is more frequent in women than in men, and the disease is often manifest during the childbearing period. Thus, pregnancy occurs in a significant number of women with MG. The effect of pregnancy on myasthenia gravis is variable. Roughly 30% of pregnant myasthenics have a remission, 30% have no change, and 40% have an exacerbation.[16] A postpartum exacerbation of the disease occurs in 30% and there are rare maternal deaths. Thus it is not possible to discern a distinct effect of pregnancy on the course of MG. However, there is a paradox hidden in these statistics. Corticosteroids are very frequently (and successfully) used to treat MG, and it was the clinical remissions in rheumatoid arthritis produced during pregnancy (or viral hepatitis) that led to the discovery of the anti-inflammatory properties of glucocorticosteroids. If pregnancy alleviates rheumatoid arthritis because of changes in corticosteroid metabolism, why doesn't pregnancy have a more beneficial effect on the course of myasthenia gravis?

Myasthenia gravis affects the outcome of pregnancy. In 314 myasthenic pregnancies, there were 38 abortions (12%), of which 14 were spontaneous and 24 were therapeutic. There were 268 live births (85%) and 8 stillbirths (3%). There were 14 neonatal deaths among the live births. Thus, there is significant fetal wastage in myasthenic pregnancies.

Neonatal myasthenia gravis consists of muscular weakness in the newborn, similar to that seen in the mother. It happens because anti-AChR antibodies of the IgG isotype will cross the placenta. Neonatal MG occurred in 47 (17.6%) of the 314 cases of myasthenic pregnancy reviewed by Plauche.[16] It is first seen 12–48 hours after birth, and lasts 10 days to 15 weeks (mean duration, 3 weeks). In general, the higher the mother's titer of anti-AChR antibody, the greater the incidence and severity of the neonatal disease.[17] Nevertheless, neither the existence nor the titer of AchR antibodies in the child predict the occurrence of neonatal MG. It is not clear why there is a delay in the appearance of symptoms, but their disappearance is a result of the metabolism of maternal antibody by the newborn. There are some suggestive data indicating that in those newborns who have clinical neonatal MG, the half-life of the AChR antibodies is particularly long. This finding brings up the interesting possibility that anti-idiotypic antibodies (of fetal origin) might bind to the AChR antibodies and regulate their metabolism or their biological blocking effects on the AChR.[18] Myasthenia gravis is apparently rare *in utero,* which is difficult to understand in view of the facilitated transport of maternal IgG to the fetus. One explanation that has been put forth to explain this is that the AChR antibody is bound by alphafetoprotein.[16] This is a provocative idea, but the addition of AFP to serum containing anti-AChR did not change the ability of these antibodies to bind to the ACh receptor.[18]

Thyroid Disease

Graves' disease, or diffuse thyrotoxicosis, is believed to be caused by circulating stimulators of receptors on the thyroid follicle cells. Of great interest is LATS (long-acting thyroid stimulator), the first known anti-receptor antibody. It is able to interact with the receptor for TSH on the thyroid follicle and to cause continuous thyroid stimulation. Congenital thyrotoxicosis is uncommon, but is thought to occur via transplacental passage of LATS, which is of the IgG isotype. However, the duration of the disease in the newborn, and the familial occurrence of a number of cases of congenital thyrotoxicosis has caused some investigators to question whether LATS transport is the only pathogenetic mechanism.[19] Neonatal hypothyroidism can occur in the offspring of mothers with Hashimoto's autoimmune thyroiditis. The syndrome is transient in the neonate and is caused by the passive transfer of TSH-binding inhibitory antibodies.[20]

Diabetes

Pregnancy and diabetes interact. Pregnancy may increase the insulin requirement of pregnant diabetics, and it may cause latent diabetics to develop overt disease. These modifications of the diabetic state are the result of changes in the intermediary metabolism of the pregnant woman, and these changes increase as pregnancy advances. The increased secretion of insulin and concomitant resistance to insulin are probably mediated through the increased secretion of pregnancy hormones from the placenta. The conceptus makes added metabolic demands on the mother as well.[21]

Early in the history of modern diabetes, a successful pregnancy in a diabetic woman was uncommon. Both maternal and fetal morbidity and mortality were high. As diabetic control became more stringent, complications of pregnancy diminished in diabetics. Nevertheless, perinatal mortality in diabetes is higher than in the general population and the increased incidence of congenital anomalies is just beginning to decrease, and spontaneous abortion rates are higher than expected.[22]

It is now recognized that type I insulin-dependent diabetes mellitus (IDDM) is a disease where genetic and autoimmune factors are very significant. There are strong HLA associations with IDDM although they are different in different ethnic and racial populations. In Caucasians, there is an increased incidence of HLA-A1, B8, DR3/4 genes in IDDM. In addition, a variety of autoimmune markers have been found, including insulitis, antibodies to islet cells, and T cells autoreactive with islet cells. However, the exact nature of the responsible autoantigen(s) is as yet unknown. Whatever the antigens may be, immune damage to islet tissue is mediated through cytokines.[23]

What the pregnancy immunologist would like to know is the effect of such immunological variables on the fetus and newborn. When the perinatal mortality in IDDM was high, it was difficult to discern any immunologic consequences to the offspring. A recent study examined the risk of developing detectable IDDM in the offspring of diabetic mothers. Somewhat surprisingly, the risk was quite low except in the group of the youngest mothers (age 15–19). Even more surprisingly, the risk of developing IDDM over the next 20 years was less if the mother (alone) was diabetic than if the father (alone) was diabetic! The authors even discuss the possibility of "a protective interaction between diabetic mother and fetus."[24] Whatever the reason, these results suggest that circulating diabetogenic immune effectors such as T cells and immunoglobulins such as anti-islet cell or anti-insulin antibodies may not be sufficient to damage the fetus or newborn.[25] In other words, the situation in IDDM is quite different from the situation in SLE or myasthenia gravis.

Systemic Maternal Autoimmune Diseases

The syndromes under this rubric include the so-called "connective tissue" or "collagen-vascular" diseases; rheumatoid arthritis, systemic lupus erythematosus, anticardiolipin syndromes, scleroderma, polyarteritis nodosa, dermato/polymyositis, and ankylosing spondylitis. A hallmark of these syndromes is that a variety of tissues are affected, often because of damage produced by actual or suspected circulating autoantibodies and/or immune complexes. Frequently, there are both broadly-reactively antibodies (such as anti-DNA) and more restricted antibodies, such as anti-erythrocyte antibodies. In addition, there may be other more fundamental abnormalities. Many immunologists believe that "behind every abnormal antibody lurks an abnormal T cell."

Rheumatoid Arthritis

The etiology and pathogenesis of rheumatoid arthritis (RA) remain obscure, even after decades of research. There are genetic susceptibilities linked to certain MHC class II specificities (HLA DR-3 and DR-4). There has always been a suspicion that a microbial agent is at fault, but none has been causally implicated. Recent work suggests that superantigens are involved in RA[26] and these are microbial in origin. This is an important area of investigation. The role of rheumatoid factors (RF), which are antibodies to autologous immunoglobulins, is also not certain. There are general correlations between the titer of rheumatoid factors(s) and disease, but there are disconcerting instances of RA without rheumatoid factors.[27]

The question of pregnancy in rheumatoid arthritis is of extraordinary interest to the immunologist. It was the recognition that pregnancy (or, in other patients, viral hepatitis) could produce a temporary remission in rheumatoid arthritis that started Hench and colleagues on the search that ended with the discovery of the anti-inflammatory properties of glucocorticoids and later with the Nobel prize.[28,29]

Case studies involving many patients with RA show that the disease improves in as many as 73% and remains the same or gets worse in 27%.[30] The improvement generally starts in the first trimester (50%), with 14% having improvement beginning in the second trimester and 6% in the third. The improvement is sustained or progressive during pregnancy, but 90% of the improved patients relapse during the postpartum period. The timing of the relapse is unpredictable and it may occur as late as 6 months after the pregnancy is over. The improvement of RA (or lack of it) in a given pregnancy is fairly predictive of the behavior of the disease in subsequent pregnancies. Thus, the response to pregnancy is stereotypic. The fetal outcome in RA is close to that seen in the general population, and spontaneous abortions occur only in severe cases.

To what can we attribute the two-thirds remission rate in women who have rheumatoid arthritis and who get pregnant? The usual answer is "hormones," but one ought to be a bit more specific. In terms of the great changes in pregnancy-associated hormonal levels, none has been proven to be responsible for the remissions in RA. Similarly, the timing of postpartum relapses has not been correlated with lactation, breast feeding, nor the reappearance of menstrual periods. Plasma cortisol levels rise, but so do corticosteroid-binding globulin levels so that clinical evidence of hypercorticism is not seen in pregnancy. None of the variables in cell-mediated immunity or T or B cell functions discussed in Chapter 2 seem like reasonable candidates. There are only sparse data about changes in rheumatoid factor titers in pregnancy. There is a suggestion that although the levels of circulating immune complexes may fall (perhaps because of binding to the placenta), the amount of IgM rheumatoid factor does not dip.[31] Recently, some sophisticated immunochemical questions have been raised. Serum IgG in RA is less glycosylated than normal IgG; in particular, it has less galactose. Pregnancy IgG, on the contrary, has more galactose associated with it. Is it possible that RA IgG is more immunogenic (leading to more RF production), whereas in pregnancy the balance shifts to less antigenic IgG?[32] In this case, the remission in pregnancy-associated RA should be correlated with a fall in RF titer, which is not a frequent finding. Nevertheless, the idea that pregnant women with RA have circulating material that is anti-inflammatory still has appeal. This idea has led to trials where nonpregnant women with RA were injected with gammaglobulin extracted from placentas. Improvement has been reported, but the trials were not controlled.[30]

Even if the improvement in RA that occurs in two-thirds of the patients when they become pregnant could be correlated with some change in hormonal or immune complex status, what about the other third who get no better or who get worse? Did those changes not occur, or were the women refractory to them? And how do we account for these patients in which rheumatoid arthritis begins in pregnancy?

In fact, we still do not know why rheumatoid arthritis often improves in pregnancy.

Systemic Lupus Erythematosus

Systemic lupus erythematosus (SLE) represents a very complicated syndrome in which there are a wide variety of immunological abnormalities. These include antibodies of broad specificity (e.g., anti-nuclear antibodies), and sometimes well-defined antibodies to specific antigens, circulating immune complexes, and perhaps some changes in the overall suppressor aspect of the immunoregulatory apparatus.[33] The disease is of interest to the pregnancy immunologist because pregnancy affects the course of SLE, because SLE affects the course and outcome of the pregnancy, and because of neonatal SLE.

Most, but not all, students of SLE believe that pregnancy is a risk factor for disease exacerbation. Because the disease waxes and wanes in the nonpregnant state, and because treatment protocols for treating SLE have changed, the subject needs reexamination from time to time. A large recent prospective study by Mintz and Rodriguez-Alvarez is pertinent.[34] They followed 102 pregnancies in 75 SLE patients. In 10 patients, the disease was considered to be active at conception and could be pharmacologically controlled early in the pregnancy. In 92 pregnancies, the disease was inactive at conception and there were 55 clinical exacerbations (60%) during the following pregnancies. Of these 55 exacerbations, 30 occurred during the first trimester, 7 in the second, 7 in the third, 9 postpartum, and 2 postabortion. Although there was not a control group of nonpregnant SLE patients who were similarly studied, most physicians would interpret the above data to indicate that pregnancy is likely to cause a disease flare in SLE.

What is the cause of these pregnancy-associated flares? A widely held opinion is that situations in which there is tissue damage, e.g., with systemic infections or following a severe sunburn, may lead to a "lupus flare" because of the release of nuclear and cytoplasmic antigens that are recognized by the already activated immune system. This, in turn, leads to increased autoantibody production and, since the tissue antigens will be present for some time, to increased titers of antigen–antibody complexes. If this is so, then it is easy to explain the lupus flares that occur postpartum; they would be provoked by the tremendous tissue damage that occurs during placental separation. However, this argument does not account for the majority of lupus flares that occur during the first trimester.

The risk to the fetus in SLE pregnancies is considerable.[35] In the series described earlier there were 17 spontaneous abortions, 50 premature deliveries, and only 35 term pregnancies.[34] Of the spontaneous abortions, 11 occurred in the first trimester and 6 in the second. Of the 50 premature deliveries, there were 5 stillbirths and one neonatal death. Thus the fetal loss (spontaneous abortions, stillbirths, and a neonatal death) was 22.5% vs 6.7% in a control set of pregnancies without SLE. (It should be noted that the control fetal loss rate is considerably lower than in many other studies.) Fetal wastage appears to be more severe when SLE is diagnosed during the pregnancy in contrast to a more benign course when SLE was present before pregnancy began.[36] However, this effect may be related to the fact that preexistent SLE can be controlled better and pregnancies can be planned in contrast to the situation where SLE declares itself *in medias res* during an ongoing pregnancy.

What are the causes of the poor fetal outcomes? One approach is to look at the placenta. Eleven patients with SLE delivered 7 live infants (three were premature) and there were 4 fetal losses between 12 and 27 weeks of gestation.[37] (All 4 were associated with anticardiolipin antibodies and thrombocytopenia in the mother.) The placentas were small and contained a variety of abnormalities including infarction, intraplacental hematomas, thickened trophoblast membranes, and deposition of immunoglobulin and complement. Another study looked at an extremely heterogeneous group of SLE patients, many on treatment, and with a variety of pregnancy outcomes.[38] Vasculitis with deposition of immunoglobulins and complement occurred in half the placentas. Taken together, these change suggest that vascular abnormalities, perhaps a true vasculitis, may result in placental insufficiency. However, adequate controls were not sufficient in these studies. Furthermore, the changes are not specific for SLE, because similar changes have been found in pre-eclampsia.[39]

Neonatal SLE is caused, perhaps exclusively, by transplacental passage of maternal antibodies. It is frequently stated that newborns with the neonatal SLE syndrome do not *really* have SLE. This means that they are suffering from passive autoimmunity and that a spontaneous active autoimmune process is not present. It does not mean that *real* immunopathologic damage does not occur.

Studies of tissue damage in neonatal SLE have focused on the skin, heart, and the hematologic systems. In a prospective study of 91 infants born to mothers with SLE, there was a 42% incidence of antinuclear antibodies in the babies; these included anti-SSA (anti-Ro), anti-SSB (anti-La), or anti-ribonucleoprotein (anti-RNP). However, only 4% of the newborns had definite neonatal SLE and another 4% had possible neonatal SLE.[40] Thus, as in adults, the mere presence of circulating antinuclear antibodies does not necessarily entail detectable autoimmune tissue damage. However, it may depend on which antibodies are present. Rare patients with neonatal SLE have been reported who have antibodies to U-RNP but not to SS-A or SS-B.[41] With regard to anticardiolipin antibodies, a prospective study showed that midpregnancy fetal distress or fetal death was closely correlated with a rise in these antibodies.[42] It is interesting that many mother-infant pairs were SS-A positive but negative on ANA screening.[43]

The cutaneous lesions of neonatal SLE resemble those in adults and are associated with the presence of anti-SSA antibodies.[44] The skin changes may not be evident immediately after delivery, and they usually resolve by 6 months.[43] Cardiac lesions include endocardial fibroelastosis and heartblock, either partial or complete.[45] A number of studies have investigated the relation of anti-SSA antibodies to heartblock, partly because of the clinical importance of the problem and partly because anti-SSA binds to cardiac tissue.[44] Ro (SSA) antigens are found in the tissues of the conducting system.[46] Neither fertility nor fetal outcome was correlated with the presence or absence of maternal anti-SSA antibodies, but both the presence and the titer of the antibody was related to congenital heartblock.[47] Nonetheless, most women with anti-SSA antibodies do not have babies with congenital heartblock[40] and there are cases where heartblock occurred without demonstrable anti-SSA.[47] It is not surprising that the prognosis of neonatal SLE is better in those with disease limited to the skin; newborns with congenital heart block do not fare as well.[48]

Finally, one might expect that babies with neonatal SLE may have hematological abnormalities. These include transient hemolytic anemia, leukopenia, and thrombocytopenia. In general these are faint reflections of similar problems in the mother and do not constitute important clinical problems.[44]

It should be pointed out that although babies with neonatal SLE can have cutaneous, cardiac, and hematologic abnormalities, they do *not* have nephritis or arthritis—two of the most characteristic lesions of active SLE itself.[44] An hypothesis that might explain this dichotomy relies on the differential passage of antibodies vs antigen–antibody complexes across the placenta. The cutaneous, cardiac, and hematological abnormalities probably represent the effects of antibodies *per se* binding to the respective target tissues. These immunoglobulins, if they are of the IgG isotype, cross the placenta. The arthritis and nephritis of SLE probably result from "innocent bystander" tissue damage, produced by the deposition of antigen–antibody complexes. In these situations, the antibodies are not directed to the synovium or the glomerular basement membrane. If these complexes are trapped in the placenta, perhaps by Fc receptors, it would explain the absence of nephritis and synovitis in neonatal SLE.

Antiphospholipid Antibody (APA) Syndromes

There has been a great deal of interest in recent years in women with antibodies to phospholipids, whether those women have known autoimmune disease or are otherwise "normal." As the field is rather new, there are some differences in laboratory techniques, in terminology, and in opinion. These problems are important in the context of this book because antiphospholipid antibodies appear to be associated with risk to both mother and fetus.

APA are detected in three basic ways. First, there is the standard flocculation test using cardiolipin antigen. When positive, it either denotes syphilitic or a similar infection, or, if these infections are not present and the test is repeatedly positive, it is called a biologically false positive (BFP) serological test for syphilis. Both retrospective and prospective studies have shown an increased incidence of autoimmune disease, particularly SLE, in people with a BFP.[49] Second, some patients with SLE were found to have prolonged partial thromboplastin times in vitro, and these sera contained material that inhibited clotting of normal blood. This phenomenon gave rise to the term, "lupus anticoagulant," (LAC). Although this term is correct in the coagulation laboratory, it is in fact a misnomer, as the clinical picture most commonly seen with LAC is thrombosis, not hemorrhage. Third, the ELISA technique was applied to the detection of antibodies to phospholipids.[50] This technique is sensitive and can be adapted to determine the phospholipid specificity of the APA and the immunoglobulin isotype.

It is clear that the BFP, LAC, and ELISA techniques do not each measure the same antiphospholipid antibodies, and in fact there may be antibodies to a variety of phospholipid antigens, all of which antibodies may not be present in a given serum. The generic term, APA, will be used here to designate positivity in any or all of the tests.

Clinically, APA can be seen in SLE and a variety of other autoimmune syndromes as well as in people without a demonstrable autoimmune disease. The primary manifestations are venous or arterial thrombosis, thrombocytopenia, and fetal loss.[51] Less frequent manifestations include a variety of vascular problems such as transient ischemic attacks, and migraine as well as chorea gravidarum and preeclampsia.[52]

It is very difficult to determine the presence and magnitude of the risks to the fetus and mother when the latter has a positive APA. One needs to take into account a panoply of variables, which are listed in Table 1, and it is desirable to evaluate the

Table 1
Antiphospholipid Antibodies[a]

1.	What APA tests were used-BFP, LAC, ELISA, or others?
2.	How sensitive are the tests and how positive are they in non-pregnant, healthy women?
3.	How high were the APA titers and how did they fluctuate during the pregnancy in question?
4.	Did the woman have a diagnosable autoimmune syndrome?
5.	Did the woman have other clinical manifestations of the APA syndrome, such as a history of thrombosis, thrombocytopenia, or neurological events, or is the APA an isolated "serological diagnosis?"
6.	Was treatment (e.g., corticosteroids) being used, and was it beneficial or even necessary?

[a]Some variables to be assessed in determining the risk to a pregnancy.

problem prospectively. To date, no study has taken all of these variables into consideration. However, a number of tentative statements may be made.

Patients with SLE have more fetal losses if they also have APA and at least one group feels that the presence of APA predicts fetal distress.[42] IgG APAs are more important than IgM APA's in predicting difficulties.[51] It is debated, however, whether the presence of a positive APA test without overt or diagnosable SLE puts a woman at greater risk for a miscarriage. In habitual aborters, retrospective analysis showed a very high incidence of IgG APA[53] but a prospective study did not.[54] There is also no unanimity about the risk of having LAC or a BFP.[55] One recent prospective study found that APAs were present in 2.2% of 737 pregnant patients, and 75% of these 16 patients had an adverse pregnancy outcome.[56] In these 16 patients, there were 8 perinatal deaths (including 4 SAbs), 4 infants with low birth weights, and 4 normal outcomes. Although authors state that the presence of a positive APA test does not invariably predict an adverse pregnancy outcome, such serological findings certainly point to a guarded prognosis. This is an impressive result.

Nevertheless, a still more recent case control study reported that in women who had not had a previous spontaneous abortion a positive APA test was not a risk factor for spontaneous abortion or fetal death.[57] This study did not consider women with repeated pregnancy losses.

The situation, I believe, can be summarized as follows:

1. SLE itself presents a risk to the fetus, and this risk is greater if APAs are detected; and
2. The presence of APAs in women who do not have a recognized autoimmune disease is less than that in SLE with APA but may be greater than that in women without APA.

The underlying basis for fetal wastage in APA syndromes may well be the same as in SLE fetal wastage, i.e., related to placental thrombosis. A variety of mechanisms have been proposed to explain the in vivo clotting abnormality seen with APA. These include changes in fibrinolytic and coagulation mechanisms, endothelial dysfunction, complement activation, and prostacycline production.[52] More than one cause may operate.

From the heuristic point of view, the antiphospholipid syndromes raise an interesting question, although not exactly a new one. Does the presence of APA in the absence of a recognizable and diagnosable autoimmune syndrome such as RA or SLE, indicate a "subclinical" autoimmune syndrome, a "pre-autoimmune" syndrome, or even a "new" autoimmune syndrome? Are these patients similar in some way to those with "serological lupus," i.e., positive serological tests for SLE without overt clinical disease?

Miscellaneous

There are a number of less common connective tissue diseases in which data about materno–fetal relations are available. The above discussion about APA should make it evident, however, that in some patients, precise diagnoses of this or that autoimmune "disease" are not always possible. One might say that the "autoimmune borders" between conditions may at times be indistinct, for instance in some patients who have some features of both SLE and scleroderma. These situations sometimes lead to the description of "overlap syndromes," a term with its own indistinct borders. It is an area that still contains uncertainties.

Scleroderma-associated pregnancies do occur, although scleroderma is more often seen in older rather than in child-bearing women. The disease is clinically heterogeneous and there may be some differences in both maternal and fetal outcome depending on whether the mother has diffuse scleroderma (progressive systemic sclerosis) or limited scleroderma (CREST syndrome—calcinosis, Raynaud's phenomenon, esophageal involvement, sclerodactyly, telangiectasias). Case reports tend to be skewed toward the unusual or the disastrous outcome, whereas comprehensive series, either retrospective or prospective, allow for more judicious opinions. With regard to the mother's disease, pregnancy produces no characteristic changes— some mothers get better, some get worse, and some are unchanged. Toxemia has been described in case reports, and is liable to lead to fatal renal failure. With regard to the fetus, several groups reported an increase in spontaneous abortion, as high as 20%. One group, however, mentioned no increase in spontaneous abortions or fetal death but instead pointed out an increased incidence of prematurity and intrauterine growth retardation.[58] The nature of the processes responsible for the fetal risk have not been clarified, but a vascular pathogenesis is likely in view of the vascular involvement so characteristic of scleroderma.[59,60] Indeed, renal failure on a vascular basis, owing to intimal proliferation, is a major cause of death in diffuse scleroderma, with or without an associated pregnancy.[58]

The etiology and pathogenesis of scleroderma remain obscure. The presence of some circulating material, perhaps toxic to endothelium, is an attractive possibility.[61] However, there are no reported cases of neonatal scleroderma. Does this mean that circulating factors are not important, or that they do not pass the placenta?

Polyarteritis nodosa (PAN) is a systemic disease characterized by arterial inflammation, sometimes with vascular occlusion or aneurysm formation. It is caused by inflammation following the deposition of antigen–antibody complexes, and thus it resembles serum sickness.[62] Although it is less common in females, some pregnancies have been reported. In 11 pregnancies, there was considerable risk to both mother and fetus. All seven mothers whose PAN began during pregnancy or postpartum died, whereas all 4 who had PAN diagnosed previously but whose disease was not active, survived.[63] There were 2 spontaneous and 2 therapeutic abortions but 7 live births, some of which were premature. Interestingly, there was one case of neonatal PAN that showed itself as a form of a transient but severe peripheral vasculitis.[64] This implies that some or all of the components of the putative circulating immune complexes passed the placenta and caused damage in the fetus. However, additional cases of neonatal PAN have not been recognized.

Dermatomyositis and polymyositis are conditions that have overlapping features and that may be combined into one term, *dermato/polymyositis* (DM/PM). The basic problem is chronic inflammation of skin and muscle, but the cause is not known. Mintz [65] has reviewed the clinical experience of DM/PM in pregnancy. In the form of the disease that begins in childhood, the symptoms flared in 4/10 pregnancies and there were 2 fetal losses. In adult DM/PM that pre-existed the pregnancy, and was in remission either spontaneously or with treatment, the disease did not become more severe and there were 5/8 live births. If, however, DM/PM appeared during pregnancy, there were only 3/8 successful pregnancies as 5 succumbed *in utero* or in the perinatal period. Interestingly, the placentas were not abnormal and neonatal DM/PM has not been reported.

Ankylosing spondylitis (AS) is an inflammatory disease primarily affecting the axial joints and very closely associated with the presence of HLA B-27.[66] It is also seen in conjunction with other putatively autoimmune conditions such as ulcerative colitis and psoriasis. Unlike rheumatoid arthritis, rheumatoid factors are almost always absent in AS. AS appears to be more frequent in males than in females, with a sex ratio of 5:1 to 9:1,[67] but there are a number of reports of pregnancy in women with AS.

Because of some similarities to rheumatoid arthritis, it is intriguing to learn what the effect of pregnancy is on the course of AS. In retrospective studies, of 131 patients assessed, 46 improved (35%), 24 deteriorated (18%), and 61 (47%) were unchanged.[68] There were 51 postpartum flares in 126 patients. In prospective studies of 27 pregnancies, 10 women had no change in their AS and 11 got worse, frequently postpartum. It is curious that the only patients who improved were the 6 who had either ulcerative colitis or psoriasis.[68]

These data are intriguing, but the correct interpretations are not obvious. Does the 35% improvement of AS in pregnancy, in contrast to the two-thirds improvement in RA, mean that there are fundamental differences in the pathogenesis of the two diseases? Does the fact that only those AS patients who also had ulcerative colitis or psoriasis improved in pregnancy mean that their diseases are fundamentally different from the other patients who had AS alone?

Graft-vs-Host Disease (GVHD)

As discussed in Chapter 1, GVHD may occur when allogeneic T cells are transferred into a host that is incapable of rejecting them, and where they react against the histocompatibility antigens of the host. It did not escape the notice of the pioneers in the field that pregnancy afforded at least a theoretical scenario in which the 3 basic requirements for GVHD are met:

1. Immunoreactive T cells from the mother reach the fetus;
2. The mother and the fetus are histoincompatible to the extent that the fetus has HLA antigens that are foreign to the mother; and
3. The fetus, being immature, is unable to destroy the mother's T cells.

Together, these conditions would allow a maternal T cell attack on the paternally-derived alloantigens on the fetus. At one point, just before the first recognized cases of GVHD (which were transfusion-related) were reported, Billingham stated that human GVHD "remains a purely theoretical hazard of pregnancy."[69]

Within the next year a case was reported in which there was XX/XY lymphoid chimerism in an infant with an immunodeficiency syndrome including thymic alymphoplasia. The patient had frequent infections, a dysgammaglobulinemia, thymic atrophy, a rash, and hepatic portal inflammation.[70] The interpretation was that this situation probably represented a case of GVHD with secondary immunologic failure, which is a regular feature of experimental GVHD. Another case with similar clinical features was claimed to represent GVHD. Although this is possible, the question of paternity and the lack of proof of maternal chimerism weaken the argument that GVHD was present in the second case.[71]

One must consider an additional possible mechanism that might lead to pregnancy-associated GVHD. If this syndrome requires some diminution of fetal anti-maternal immunoreactivity, this situation could also exist for genetic reasons, and be specifically related to the mother. The senario would be analogous to the experiments in inbred animals where parental (A x A)T cells are injected into (A X C)F1 recipients. GVHD ensues, even if the recipient is unsuppressed. Parental T cells recognize and react against the MHC antigens on the F1 recipient encoded by the C genes. The F1 in turn bears the MHC-A gene products and is thus incapable of rejecting the donor T cells that are seen as "self." This special situation favoring GVHD would be very different if the mother were heterozygous (e.g., A X D). In this case, maternal cells bearing A and D MHC antigens would be recognized as foreign and would be destroyed by the fetus by virtue of their having the D antigens that are "not-self" to the fetus.

With this in mind, consider a situation in which a mother is homozygous at one or more HLA loci. This leads to a situation where her T cells will be able to react against the paternally-

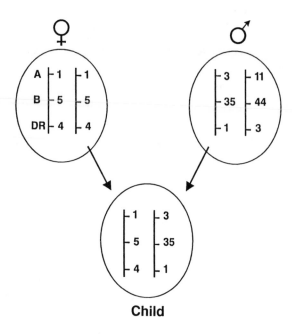

Child

Fig. 1. In this situation, mother is homozygous for HLA-A1, B5, DR4. Thus, although she would be able to react to the paternal antigens on the fetus (HLA-A3, B35, DR1), the fetus would not be able to react against the maternal cells, as their HLA would be seen as "self" by the fetal immune system.

derived HLA antigens on the fetus but the fetus will not react against the maternal T cells because the homozygous HLA gene products will be seen as "self." Thus we would have GVHD without a corresponding HVG (host-vs-graft) reaction. The situation is outlined in Fig. 1.

There are data indicating that there is increased HLA-DR compatibility between parent and child in severe combined immunodeficiency (SCID) and other neonatal hematopoietic diseases.[72] These data raise the possibility that instances of SCID where there is no clear autosomal recessive inheritance might represent the outcome of GVHD. This situation is illustrated by a child with immunodeficiency and GVHD, the latter being manifest not only by a clinical picture consistent with GVHD but with persistent circulating activated maternal T cells. The mother was homozygous at the A, B, and DR loci and her activated T cells in the fetus were most likely reacting against paternal antigens. It is intriguing that, in spite of continued maternal T cell chimerism, the GVHD symptoms disappeared with time, perhaps because of the development of suppressor cells.[73] A larger series described 16 infants with SCID. Four had circulating maternal T cells but clinical GVHD was not severe.[74] The interpretation of these data was that some cases of SCID may be caused by intrauterine GVHD, but that maternal T cell chimerism may not necessarily presage fatal GVHD.

Finally, an immunologic engineering approach was tried so as to eliminate the maternal cells (graft #1) persisting in SCID and causing GVHD. This was done by introducing a graft-vs-graft situation in which a bone marrow graft (graft #2) from an HLA-identical sibling was given to a child with SCID and GVHD. This resulted in a temporary exacerbation of the GVHD, but the development of active CTLs leading to the elimination of maternal T cells (graft #1).[75]

Other maternofetal incompatibilities may be involved. A case of maternal isoimmunization to platelet antigens apparently led to SCID and fatal GVHD.[7] The hypothesis was that isoimmunization led to impairment of the fetal immune system. In this case, there was considerable HLA sharing in the parents and the persistence of maternal T cells in the newborn established the existence of chimerism as a basis for GVHD.

Thus, pregnancy-associated GVHD exists and appears to be favored by maternal homozygosity and the presence of fetal immunoincompetence, e.g., SCID. However, the interrelations between immunoincompetence permitting maternal cells to cause GVHD, and maternally-induced GVHD leading to fetal incompetence have not yet been fully explored.

Materno–Fetal Interaction that Might Be Immunlogically Mediated

There are conditions not yet completely understood, where immune processes might be important. These include the pre-eclamptic syndromes and repeated spontaneous abortion. The latter will be discussed separately in Chapter 6.

Pre-eclampsia (PE) is a condition in which the extravillous trophoblast fails to invade the spiral arteries of the myometrium, leading to a failure of the development of a low-resistance vascular system.[76] There is vascular hyperreactivity and a clinical picture dominated by maternal gestational hypertension often accompanied by excessive edema and/or proteinuria.[77]

As with most diseases of unknown cause, there is a broad list of possible etiologies, including various immunologic processes.[76,78] In spite of a list of candidate causes, this observer is not certain that significant progress has been made in pinning down any of the causes of preeclampsia in the last 40 years.

Nevertheless, there are tantalizing clinical observations in preeclampsia that need to be considered in any etiologic or pathogenetic schema. Some data favor a genetic hypothesis, such as the study that found a 26% incidence of PE in daughters of women with PE but only an 8% incidence in the daughters-in-law.[79] Immunologists (and others) have been intrigued by the fact that PE is at least twice as frequent in first than in subsequent pregnancies. Several correlations have been made to try to account for the decreased incidence of PE in second and later pregnancies. One study indicated that the "protective effect" required that the first pregnancy last at least 37 weeks.[80] A very large retrospective survey of almost 30,000 deliveries indicated that even a previous abortion slightly but significantly decreased the incidence of PE from 25.4 to 22.3% ($p < 0.01$) but a previous term pregnancy was more protective, lowering the frequency of PE to 10%. (The effect of changing partners was not studied.[81]) The protective effect of a prior term pregnancy is well known, but the smaller protective effect of a prior miscarriage would not have been seen had the number of patients been less large.

It has been argued that a prior pregnancy is protective only if the father was the same in both pregnancies. In a large survey of women who had PE following at least one previous normotensive pregnancy, there was a much higher incidence than expected of having a different partner in the PE pregnancy.[82] This has given rise to the idea that there is a "father-specific" factor of some kind in preeclampsia. In a widely quoted paper supporting this idea. Need[83] cites a woman who had twins in her first pregnancy and PE in her next pregnancy with a different partner. This is just a case report, but it illustrates the model. It also points out a rather extraordinary fact in this report. Although the HLA typing methods were not as satisfactory at that time as one would like, it appears that the first father and the mother shared a considerable number of HLA antigens, whereas the mother and the second father did not. This situation was confirmed in MLR testing, where the mother's cells reacted 8 times more vigorously to the second father's cells than to the first father's cells. These results are difficult to evaluate without a large number of controls, but they do not indicate any *less* histocompatibility between the pre-eclamptic woman and her partner (the second husband). In fact, the results suggest that the HLA sharing in the first pregnancy was of such a magnitude that the pregnancy provided little if any immunologic stimulus. In other words, the *second* pregnancy was (from the immunologic standpoint) like a first pregnancy! However, this concept is opposed to data showing that couples with pre-eclampsia share *more* HLA antigens than do control couples.[84]

The possibility of a "father specific" factor is supported by isolated situations, such as the one where two women had PE, and were married to the same man (at different times).[85]

A recent report evaluated the question somewhat differently. A retrospective case controlled study confirmed an earlier paper and indicated that there was a 2.37-fold increased risk of PE in women who used birth control methods that decreased their exposure to sperm.[86] This result indicates that there is a PE-protective effect of sperm contacts. The data do not implicate any mechanism, but immunologic or not, they are intriguing, as are the data indicating that the incidence of PE is considerably less if the primigravidas had prior blood transfusions.[87]

More direct approaches to identify an immunologic etiology have been disappointing.[88] Two groups failed to find evidence for circulating antigen–antibody complexes.[89,90] A preliminary report suggested that pre-eclampsia is associated with maternal and paternal immunological hyporesponsiveness, but this finding has not been substantiated with newer cellular immunological techniques.[91] A very recent paper indicated that CD4[+] T helper cells were statistically lower before preeclampsia developed (27.0 vs 34.7% in normal pregnancy, $p < 0.001$).[92] Whether this statistical difference reflects an important biological mechanism awaits confirmation and further research. An immunological study of the infiltrate in the decidua in PE showed no important differences from normal term deciduas. It is interesting that in both cases, PE and in normal pregnancy, CTLs had little if any IL-2 receptors, again suggesting that T cell immunological regulation may be different in the placenta compared with the peripheral lymphoid tissues.[93] Finally, genetic factors may be important, as there are certain families in which PE seems to be more frequent than one would expect.[94] However, the study was retrospective and no data on HLA antigens were given.

In effect, the concept that some immunologic process(es) may underlie preeclampsia is one worth considering, but the data available so far are not compelling.

Summary

Immunologically-mediated diseases originating in the mother may affect the fetus. Conversely, the occurrence of pregnancy may alter the course of autoimmunity in the mother.

1. Maternal sensitization may develop to fetal material such as Rh, ABO, and platelet antigens.

    a. If maternal IgG is made, it can cross the placenta and affect the fetus.

    b. The development of knowledge about Rh isosensitization represents the successive recognition, explication, treatment, and now prevention of this syndrome.

2. Organ-specific maternal autoimmune diseases in the pregnant woman more often affect the fetus than the mother or the autoimmune process itself.

    a. Autoantibodies traversing the placenta may injure fetal tissue as in myasthenia gravis, and autoimmune thyroid disease.

    b. Some autoimmune processes have less effect on the fetus, such as thrombocytopenia and diabetes.

3. Systemic maternal autoimmune disease in which pregnancy occurs includes a variety of connective tissue disorders.

    a. Rheumatoid arthritis is the outstanding example of the beneficial effects of pregnancy on autoimmunity. RA is not, however, improved in every pregnancy, and the mechanism by which improvement occurs is still unknown.

    b. SLE in pregnancy is associated with significant increase in disease severity in the mother and with fetal wastage.

    c. Anti-phospholipid antibody (APA) syndromes present a recently-noticed pregnancy hazard. It is not clear whether the presence of APL antibodies is a separate form of autoimmunity, but increased fetal loss is associated with these syndromes.

4. Graft-vs-host disease may occur if immunocompetent maternal T cells react against fetal alloantigens.

    a. This situation is infrequent and is favored by homozygosity in the mother, and possibly by severe combined immunodeficiency in the fetus.

5. Pre-eclamsia has not been proven to have important immunologic aspects to its pathogenesis but there are some tantalizing clues available.

References

1. Levine P, Katzin EM, Burnham L: Isoimmunization in pregnancy: It's possible bearing on the etiology of erythroblastosis fetalis. *JAMA* 1941; 116: 825–827.

2. Konugres AA: Non-Rh hemolytic disease of the newborn, in Bern MM, Frigoletto FDJ (eds): *Hematologic Disorders in Maternal Fetal Medicine.* New York, NY, Wiley-Liss; 1990: 153–169.

3. Taaning E, Skibsted L: The frequency of platelet alloantibodies in pregnant women and the occurrence and management of neonatal alloimmune thrombocytopenic purpura. *Obstet Gynecol Surv* 1990; 45: 521–525.

4. Marcus DM, Kundu SK, Suzuki A: The P blood group system: Recent progress in immunochemistry and genetics. *Semin Hematol* 1981; 18: 63–71.

5. Deaver JE, Leppert PC, Zaroulis CG: Neonatal alloimmune thrombocytopenic purpura. *Am J Perinatol* 1986; 3: 127–131.

6. Blanchette VS: Neonatal alloimmune thrombocytopenia, in Stockman JAIII, Pochedly C (eds): *Developmental and Neonatal Hematology.* New York, Raven Press; 1988: 145–168.

7. Bastian JF, Williams RA, Ornelas W, et al.: Maternal iso-immunization resulting in combined immunodeficiency and fatal graft-versus-host disease in an infant. *Lancet* 1984; i: 1435–1437.

8. Shornick JK, Bangert JL, Freeman RG, et al.: Herpes gestationis: Clinical and histologic features of twenty-eight cases. *J Am Acad Dermatol* 1983; 8: 214–224.

9. Chorzelski TP, Jablouska S, Beutner EH, et al.: Herpes gestations with identical lesions in the newborn: Passive transfer of the disease? *Arch Dermatol* 1976; 112: 1129–1131.

10. Lookingbill DP, Chez RA: Herpes gestationis. *Clin Obstet Gynecol* 1983; 26: 605–614.

11. Shornick JK, Stastny P, Gilliam JN: High frequency of histocompatibility antigens HLA-DR3 and DR4 in herpes gestationis. *J Clin Invest* 1981; 68: 553–555.

12. Cines DB, Dusak B, Tomask A, et al.: Immune thrombocytopenic purpura and pregnancy. *N Engl J Med* 1982; 306: 826–831.

13. O'Reilly R, Taber B: Immunologic thrombocytopenic purpura and pregnancy. *Obstet Gynecol* 1978; 51: 590–597.

14. Sokol RJ, Hewitt S, Stamps BK: Erythrocyte autoantibodies, autoimmune hemolysis and pregnancy. *Vox Sang* 1982; 43: 169–176.

15. Rose JW, McFarlin DE: Myasthenia gravis, in Samter M, Talmage DW, Frank MM, Austen KF, Claman HN (eds): *Immunological Diseases*. Boston, Little, Brown & Co.; 1988: 1851–1875.

16. Plauche WC: Myasthenia gravis. *Clin Obstet Gynecol* 1983; 26: 592–604.

17. Morel E, Eymard B, Vernet der Garabedian B, et al.: Neonatal myasthenia gravis: A new clinical and immunologic appraisal on 30 cases. *Neurology* 1986; 38: 138–142.

18. Lefvert AK, Osterman PO: Newborn infants to myasthenic mothers: A clinical study and investigation of acetylcholine receptor antibodies in 17 children. *Neurology* 1983; 33: 133–138.

19. Hollingsworth DR, Mabroy CC: Congenital Grave's disease: Four familial cases with long-term follow-up and perspective. *Am J Dis Child* 1976; 130: 149–155.

20. Matsuura N, Yamada Y, Nohara Y, et al.: Familial neonatal transient hypothyroidism due to maternal TSH-binding inhibitor immunoglobulins. *N Engl J Med* 1980; 303: 738.

21. Metzger BE, Frienkel N: Pregnancy complicated by diabetes mellitus, in DeGroot LJ (ed): *Endocrinology*. Philadelphia, W. B. Saunders Co.; 1989: 1408–1423.

22. Coustan DR, Felig P: Diabetes mellitus, in Burrow GN, Ferris TF (eds): *Medical Complications During Pregnancy*. Philadelphia, W. B. Saunders Co.; 1988: 34–64.

23. Mandrup-Poulsen T, Nerup J: The autoimmune hypothesis of insulin-dependent diabetes: 1965 to the present, in Ginsberg-Fellner F, McEvoy RC (eds): *Autoimmunity and the Pathogenesis of Diabetes*. New York, Springer-Verlag; 1990: 1–28.

24. Warram JH, Martin BC: Possible mechanisms for the diminished risk of IDDM in the children of diabetic mothers, in Andreani D, Bompiani G, DiMario U, Faulk WP, Galluzo A (eds): *Immuno-biology of Normal and Diabetic Pregnancy*. New York, Wiley; 1990: 221–230.

25. Giordano C: Immunobiology of normal and diabetic pregnancy. *Immunol Today* 1990; 11: 301–303.

26. Paliard X, West SG, Lafferty JA, et al.: Evidence for the effects of a superantigen in rheumatoid arthritis. *Science* 1991; 253: 325–329.

27. Good RA, Rotstein J, Mozzitello WF: The simultaneous occurrence of rheumatoid arthritis and agammaglobulinemia. *J Lab Clin Med* 1957; 49: 343–357.

28. Hench PS: The ameliorating effect of pregnancy on chronic atrophic (infectious rheumatoid) arthritis, fibrosis, and intermitteny hydrarthosis. *Proc Staff Mtgs Mayo Clin* 1938; 13: 161–167.

29. Hench PS: The reversibility of certain rheumatic and non-rheumatic conditions by the use of cortisone or of the pituitary adrenocorticotrophic hormone. *Ann Int Med* 1952; 36: 1–38.

30. Klipple G, Cecere FA: Rheumatoid arthritis and pregnancy. *Rheum Dis Clinics N Am* 1989; 15: 213–239.

31. Pope RM, Yoshinoya S, Rutstein J, et al.: Effect of pregnancy on immune complexes and rheumatoid factors in patients with rheumatoid arthritis. *Am J Med* 1983; 74: 973–979.

32. Stanworth D: A possible immunochemical explanation for pregnancy associated remissions in rheumatoid arthritis? *Ann Rheum Dis* 1988; 47: 89–90.

33. Klinman DM, Steinberg AD: Systemic lupus erythematosus and overlap syndromes, in Samter M, Talmage DW, Frank MM, Austen KF, Claman HN (eds): *Immunological Diseases*. Boston, Little, Brown & Co.; 1988: 1335–1364.

34. Mintz G, Rodriguez-Alvarez E: Systemic lupus erythematosus. *Rheum Dis Clinics N Am* 1989; 15: 255–274.

35. Englert HJ, Derve GM, Loizou S, et al.: Pregnancy and lupus: Prognostic indicators and response to treatment. *Q J Med* 1988; 250: 125–136.

36. Bobrie G, Liote F, Houillier P, et al.: Pregnancy in lupus nephritis and related disorders. *Am J Kidney Dis* 1987; 9: 339–343.

37. Hanly JG, Gladman DD, Rose TH, et al.: Lupus pregnancy: A prospective study of placental changes. *Arth Rheum* 1988; 31: 358–366.

38. Abramowsky CR, Vegas ME, Swinehart G, et al.: Decidual vasculopathy of the placenta in lupus erythematosus. *N Engl J Med* 1980; 303: 668–672.

39. Kitzmiller JL, Benirschke K: Immunofluorescent study of placental bed vessels in pre-eclampsia of pregnancy. *Am J Obstet Gynecol* 1973; 115: 248–251.

40. Lockshin MD, Bonfa E, Elkon K, et al.: Neonatal lupus risk to newborns of mothers with systemic lupus erythematosus. *Arth Rheum* 1988; 31: 697–701.
41. Provost TT, Watson R, Gammon WR, et al.: The neonatal lupus syndrome associated with U1RNP (nRNP) antibodies. *N Engl J Med* 1987; 316: 1135–1138.
42. Lockshin MD, Druzin ML, Goei S, et al.: Antibody to cardiolipin as a predictor of fetal distress or death in pregnant patients with systemic lupus erythematosus. *N Engl J Med* 1985; 313: 152–156.
43. Watson RM, Lane AT, Barnett NK, et al.: Neonatal lupus erythematosus: A clinical serological and immunogenetic study with review of the literature. *Medicine* 1984; 63: 362–378.
44. Goldsmith DP: Neonatal rheumatic disorders: View of the pediatrician. *Rheum Dis Clinics N Am* 1989; 15: 287–305.
45. McCue CM, Mantakas ME, Tinglestad JB, et al.: Congenital heart block in newborns of mothers with connective tissue disease. *Circulation* 1977; 56: 82–90.
46. Henley WL: Autoimmunity and autoimmune diseases, in Sweet AY, Brown EG (eds): *Fetal and Neonatal Effects of Maternal Disease*. Mosby; 1991: 378–391.
47. Ramsey-Goldman R, Hom D, Deng JS, et al.: Anti-SS-A antibodies and fetal outcome in maternal systemic lupus erythematosus. *Arth Rheum* 1986; 29: 1269–1273.
48. McCune AB, Weston WL, Lee LA: Maternal and fetal outcome in neonatal lupus erythematosus. *Ann Int Med* 1987; 106: 518–523.
49. Moore JE, Jutz WB: The natural history of systemic lupus erythematosus: An approach to its study through chronic biologic false positive reactors. *J Chron Dis* 1955; 1: 297–316.
50. Harris EN, Gharan AE, Boey ML, et al.: Anticardiolipin antibodies: Detection by radioimmunoassay and association with thrombosis in systemic lupus erythematosus. *Lancet* 1983; 2: 1211–1214.
51. Harris EN, Chan JKH, Asherson RA, et al.: Thrombosis, recurrent fetal loss and thrombocytopenia: Predictive value of the anticardiolipin antibody test. *Arch Intern Med* 1986; 146: 2153–2156.

52. Branch DW: Antiphospholipid antibodies and pregnancy: Maternal implications. *Semin Perinatol* 1990; 14: 139–146.

53. Unander AM, Norberg R, Hahn L, et al.: Anticardiolipin antibodies and complement in ninety-nine women with habitual abortion. *Am J Obstet Gynecol* 1987; 156: 114–119.

54. Petri M, Golbus M, Anderson R, et al.: Antinuclear antibody, lupus anticoagulant and anticardiolipin antibody in women with idiopathic habitual abortion: A controlled, prospective study of forty-four women. *Arthritis Rheum* 1987; 30: 601–606.

55. Parke AL: Antiphospholipid antibody syndromes. *Rheum Dis Clinics N Am* 1989; 15: 275–286.

56. Lockwood CJ, Romero R, Feinberg RF, et al.: The prevalence and biological significance of lupus anticoagulant and anti-cardiolipin antibodies in a general obstetric population. *Am J Obstet Gynecol* 1989; 161: 369–373.

57. Infante-Rivard C, David D, Gauthier R, et al.: Lupus anti-coagulants, anticardiolipin antibodies, and fetal loss: A case-control study. *N Engl J Med* 1991; 325: 1063–1066.

58. Black CM, Stevens WM: Scleroderma. *Rheum Dis Clinics N Am* 1989; 15: 193–212.

59. Claman HN: On scleroderma: mast cells, endothelial cells, and fibrosis. *JAMA* 1989; 262: 1206–1209.

60. Campbell PM, LeRoy EC: Pathogenesis of systemic sclerosis: a vascular hypothesis. *Semin Arthritis Rheum* 1975; 4: 351–368.

61. Silver RM, LeRoy EC: Systemic sclerosis (scleroderma), in Samter M, Talmage DW, Frank MM, Austen KF, Claman HN (eds): *Immunological Diseases*. Boston, Little, Brown & Co.; 1988: 1459–1499.

62. Katz P, Fauci AS: Systemic vasculitis, in Samter M, Talmage DW, Frank MM, Autsen FK, Claman HN (eds): *Immunological Diseases*. Boston, Little, Brown & Co.; 1988: 1417–1436.

63. Klipple GL, Riordan KK: Rare inflammatory and hereditary connective tissue diseases. *Rheum Dis Clinics N Am* 1989; 15: 383–398.

64. Boren RJ, Everett MA: Cutaneous vasculitis in mother and infant. *Arch Dermatol* 1965; 92: 568–570.

65. Mintz G: Dermatomyositis. *Rheum Dis Clinics N Am* 1989; 15: 375–382.

66. Khan MA, Skosey JL: Ankylosing spondylitis and related spondyloarthropathies, in Samter M, Talmage DW, Frank MM, Austen KF, Claman HN (eds): *Immunological Diseases.* Boston, Little, Brown & Co.; 1988: 1509–1538.

67. Marks SH, Barnett M, Calin A: Ankylosing spondylitis in women and men: A case-control study. *J Rheumatol* 1983; 10: 624–628.

68. Ostensen M, Husby G: Ankylosing spondylitis and pregnancy. *Rheum Dis Clinics N Am* 1989; 15: 241–254.

69. Billingham RE: Transplantation immunity and the materno-fetal relation. *N Engl J Med* 1964; 270: 720–725.

70. Kadowaki J, Thompson RI, Zuelzer WW, et al.: XX/XY lymphoid chimaerism in congenital immunological deficiency syndrome with thymic alymphoplasia. *Lancet* 1965; ii: 1152–1156.

71. Grogan TM, Broghton DD, Doyle WF: Graft-versus-host reaction (GVHR): A case report suggesting GVHR occurred as a result of maternofetal cell transfer. *Arch Pathol* 1975; 99: 330–334.

72. Hansen JA, Good RA, DuPont B: HLA-D compatibility between parent and child: Increased occurrence in severe combined immunodeficiency and other hematopoietic diseases. *Transplantation* 1977; 23: 366–374.

73. Pollack MS, Kapoor N, Sorell M, et al.: DR-positive maternal engrafted T cells in a severe combined immunodeficiency patient without graft-versus-host disease. *Transplantation* 1980; 30: 331–334.

74. Pollack MS, Kirkpatrick D, Kapoor N, et al.: Identification by HLA typing of intrauterine-derived maternal T cells in four patients with severe combined immunodeficiency. *N Engl J Med* 1982; 307: 662–666.

75. le Deist F, Raffoux C, Griscelli C, et al.: Graft vs graft reaction resulting in the elimination of maternal cells in a SCID patient with maternofetal GVHD after HLA identical bone marrow transplantation. *J Immunol* 1987; 138: 423–427.

76. Clark DA: On preeclampsia and leukocytes in human decidua. *Am J Reprod Immunol* 1987; 15: 9–11.

77. MacGillivray I: *Pre-eclampsia: The hypertensive disease of pregnancy*, London, W.B. Saunders; 1983:

78. Beer AE: Immunology, contraception, and preeclampsia. *JAMA* 1989; 262: 3184–3180.

79. Chesley LC, Annitto JE, Cosgrove RA: The familial factor in toxemiae of pregnancy. *Obstet Gynecol* 1968; 32: 303–311.

80. Campbell D, MacGillivray I, Carr-Hill P: Pre-eclampsia in second pregnancy. *Br J Obstet Gynaecol* 1985; 92: 131–140.

81. Strickland DM, Guzik DS, Cox K, et al.: The relationship between abortion in the first pregnancy and development of pregnancy-induced hypertension in the subsequent pregnancy. *Am J Obstet Gynecol* 1986; 154: 146–148.

82. Feeney JG, Scott JS: Pre-eclampsia and changed paternity. *Eur J Obstet Gynecol Reprod Biol* 1980; 11: 35–38.

83. Need J: Pre-eclampsia in pregnancy by different fathers. *Br Med J* 1975; i: 548–549.

84. Jenkins DM, Need JA, Scott JS, et al.: Human leukocyte antigen and mixed lymphocyte reaction in severe pre-eclampsia. *Br Med J* 1978; i: 542–544.

85. Astin M, Scott JR, Worley RJ: Preeclampsia-eclampsia: A fatal father factor. *Lancet* 1981; ii: 533.

86. Klonoff-Cohen HS, et al.: An epidemiologic study of contraception and preeclampsia. J*AMA* 1989; 262: 3143–3140.

87. Feeney JG, Tovey LA, Scott JS: Influence of previous blood transfusion on incidence of preeclampsia. *Lancet* 1977; i: 874–875.

88. Stirrat GM: Possible role of trophoblast in preeclampsia, in Chaouat G (ed): *The Immunology of the Fetus.* Baco Raton, CRC Press, Inc.; 1990: 241–252.

89. Knox GE, Stagno S, Volanakis JE, et al.: A search for antigen-antibody complexes in pre-eclamsia: Further evidence against immunologic pathogenesis. *Am J Obstet Gynecol* 1978; 132: 87–89.

90. Balasch J, Mirapeix E, Borche L, et al.: Further evidence against preeclampsia as an immune complex disease. Obstet Gynecol 1981; 58: 435–437.

91. Birkeland SA, Kristofferson K: Pre-eclampsia: a state of mother-fetal immune imbalance. *Lancet* 1979; ii: 720–723.

92. Bardeguez AD, McNerney R, Frieri M, et al.: Cellular immunity in preeclampsia: Alterations in T-lymphoycte subpopulations during early pregnancy. *Obstet Gynecol* 1991; 77: 859–862.

93. Khong TY: An immunohistologic study of the leukocyte infiltrate in maternal uterine tissues in normal and pre-eclamptic pregnancies at term. *Am J Reprod Immunol Microbiol* 1987; 15: 1–8.

94. Cooper D: Genetic control of susceptibility to eclampsia and miscarriage. *Br J Obstet Gynaecol* 1988; 95: 644–653.

Chapter 6

Recurrent Pregnancy Loss

Immunologic and Nonimmunologic Aspects

No aspect of the immunology of pregnancy is more controversial than the subject of recurrent pregnancy loss, or, as it will be called here, recurrent spontaneous abortion (RSAb). Nor is there any subject in this book more laden with emotion because the immunologic facts, as perceived, have a very strong influence on therapy decisions for RSAb and thus, potentially, on the ability of the childless to have children. Indeed, it is the question of the relevance of immunology to RSAb that prompted the writing of this book. Because of these two factors—the controversial nature of the data and the emotional implications of the interpretation of the data—there will be few general statements in this chapter that will not be questioned by someone.

Recurrent Spontaneous Abortion

Definitions

A spontaneous abortion may be defined as the noninduced early loss of a pregnancy. By definition, it is a loss that occurs before the time at which the delivered pregnancy might be viable. (A loss at a later time would be a stillbirth.) As perinatal care has improved, younger and younger infants have survived, so that the point of viability has occurred earlier in pregnancy. One current definition states that an abortion involves the loss of a fetus/embryo of 500 g wt or less, roughly at 20–22 weeks of gestation.[1]

The definition of a "recurrent spontaneous aborter" or an "habitual aborter" is less certain. The definition usually indicates a woman who has had 3 or more spontaneous abortions, regardless of cause. The precision of this and other related definitions is very important, as they are used to guide the design of treatment protocols and the interpretation of data. Although all definitions are arbitrary, some may be more standard and more useful than others. Therefore, it is important to note that at least one group has recently stated that RSAb means 2 or more early pregnancy losses,[2] and it has been stated that "in practice," many physicians consider that two early losses denote the habitual aborter condition.[1]

It would be wise to go back one step to note the main reason underlying the importance of a clear definition of RSAb. The definition signals the transition between the "normal state," where a miscarriage, or perhaps two, is unfortunate but that does not apparently prejudice the occurrence of successful pregnancies later on, and the "abnormal state," where X number of miscarriages means "something is wrong here," and, without an investigation and perhaps treatment of some condition, future pregnancies are likely to be similarly disastrous. Where one puts the border between normality and pathology turns out to be a difficult task. It is primarily a statistical task, yet the underlying assumption is that the real biological problems underlying RSAb are different from those accounting for occasional or sporadic miscarriages.

The Frequency of Miscarriages

One very important ingredient of the definition of RSAb is a determination of the incidence of miscarriages in random pregnancies. A widely quoted statistic is that 15% of clinically recognized pregnancies end in miscarriage.[3] Recent data have been gathered using extremely sensitive hormonal measurements to detect the presence (and the loss) of very early pregnancies, even before implantation.[4,5] Both primiparas and multiparas were studied. The results confirmed what many people have believed, i.e., that many early pregnancies are lost before their presence was suspected by the usual clinical criteria. For instance, 15% of fertilized ova (very early pregnancies) were lost before implantation, and another 22% of implanted embryos (early pregnancies) were lost before it was possible to confirm a pregnancy by clinical criteria. These figures contrast strongly with a 9% loss of *clinically* confirmed pregnancies in the study. Thus, more than 3 times as many clinically inapparent pregnancies are lost compared with clinically apparent pregnancies.

If these results are projected onto the general population of women capable of becoming pregnant, it is obvious that many "primigravidas" and even "nulligravidas" will have, in fact, lost one or more early or very early pregnancies that were undetected.

These considerations become critical when evaluating the status of aborting women. If, by definition, an habitual aborter has had 3 or more miscarriages, would these very early pregnancy losses (biochemically confirmed but not clinically evident) "count"? Or do only clinically apparent pregnancy losses "count"? What we want to know is which pregnancies losses are pertinent to any possible immunological cause of RSAb and which are not. It would be naive to suppose that all pregnancy losses, from very early to early to clinically confirmed, have the same spectrum of causes.[6] Unfortunately, we do not have enough information to answer these questions, although it is believed that the earlier the abortion, the more likely it is to be chromosomally abnormal.[3] It should be noted, however, that virtually all clinical studies on RSAbs have paid attention only to clinically recognized pregnancy losses.

Primary and Secondary
Recurrent Spontaneous Abortion

An additional nosological problem arises with regard to RSAb. Some investigators make a sharp distinction between "primary" and "secondary" aborters.[7,8] A primary recurrent spontaneous aborter has had 3 (or even just 2) or more clinical miscarriages without a live baby. A secondary recurrent spontaneous aborter has had 3 or more clinical miscarriages but has had a live baby.

According to one group, primary aborting couples show more HLA sharing than do secondary aborting couples. Primary aborting women have no lymphocytotoxic antibodies or antibody-dependent cellular cytotoxicity (ADCC) against paternal antigens, whereas most secondary aborters have both of these factors.[8] However, the HLA sharing schema is not clearcut, as there are data showing that primary aborters have an increased degree of sharing at the HLA-A, B, and DR loci but secondary aborters have increased DQ sharing.[9] Furthermore, it has been stated that a primary aborter can have a successful pregnancy with a different partner whereas a secondary aborter will most likely fail with any partner.[7] These ideas are interesting, i.e., that primary abortion is immunological, reflecting problems between a particular woman and a particular man, but secondary abortion mainly reflects only a maternal problem, either genetic or autoimmune. However, firm data with regard to these prognoses are difficult to find. One retrospective study of RSAb found that the next pregnancy showed an increased incidence of low birth weight, SGA babies, and prematurity (compared with historical controls) but there was no difference in success between primary and secondary aborters.[10] Another view, however, is that the prognosis is far better with secondary aborters than with primary aborters.[11]

Paternal considerations are also important in definitions of RSAb, and geneticists and endocrinologists, for instance, view these variables differently from immunologists. If one is focusing on a maternal genetic or hormonal problem in an habitually aborting woman, whether the father of all the pregnancies is the same may be irrelevant. This may also be true for the pregnancy immunologist who is studying the effects of an autoimmune condition in the mother. But if one is considering those cases where known maternal abnormalities are not apparent, then it is presumably the relation between the woman and a specific man that is important. So the definition of RSAb and primary and secondary RSAb generally stipulate that the father is the same for all pregnancies coming under that rubric. The pregnancy history of the woman with RSAb who has had a different partner at some other time is a very intriguing but separate question. Unfortunately, it has not been systematically examined.

The Prognosis in RSAb

The prognosis in RSAb becomes a critical ingredient in the assessment of the impact of various causes of miscarriage, e.g., anatomic, genetic, and so on. It is equally critical in the assessment of the efficacy of immunological (or other) treatments for RSAb because the prognosis of (untreated) RSAb determines "the denominator" or the placebo rate in any trial.

If one considers primary aborters, the incidence of a first clinical pregnancy loss in unselected pregnant women was 15%; of first and second pregnancy losses was 2.3%; of first, second, and third pregnancy losses was 0.34%; and of losses in 1 through 4 pregnancies, 0.05%.[1] Thus, 3 losses without a successful pregnancy will occur in 34 of 10,000 women who have 3 pregnancies.

In practice, however, both the physician and the patient view the problem in a different way. They want to know "what are the chances?" in the next pregnancy. Estimates vary widely, but a summary of available data indicates that after 1 miscarriage, the risk of a second miscarriage is 13–26%; after 2 miscarriages, the risk of a third is 17–35%; and after 3 losses, the risk of a fourth is 25–46%.[12] Recently, more careful attention to this problem has produced more reliable statistics. A small prospective study from The Netherlands showed that after 3 or more spontaneous abortions, both primary and secondary aborters had a 50% success rate on the next pregnancy.[13] A very large retrospective analysis of the Danish Patient Registry had 300,500 pregnancies available for study. The abortion risk was 11% where there were no previous miscarriages, 16% after one abortion, and 25, 45, and 54% after 2, 3, and 4 abortions, respectively.[14] Taking these and previous studies together, it appears that the success rate after 3 miscarriages is about 50% in the next pregnancy.

At least two points need to be made. These statistics show that pregnancy losses in these patients are not random; if they were, the chances of a subsequent loss would be the same after 1, 2, or 3 miscarriages. Thus, there is some underlying cause(s) predisposing toward further losses. In addition, a success rate of 50% in the next clinical pregnancy, even after 3 consecutive miscarriages, must be weighed carefully when considering intervention trials.

Leaving aside the problem of the underestimation of early pregnancy losses, one wonders whether the *ordering* of the pregnancies in secondary aborters is of any relevance. Using 0 for a miscarriage and 1 for a live baby, is there any difference in pathogenesis or prognosis depending on whether the pregnancy history is 0, 0, 0, 1, compared with 1, 0, 0, 0, or even with 0, 0, 1, 0? Are these histories equivalent, and if not, how do they differ? In most reported series, these distinctions are not made, but one summary indicates that there is no significant difference in prognosis between secondary aborters where the first pregnancy was successful vs those in which *any* pregnancy was successful.[1]

Conditions Associated
with Recurrent Spontaneous Abortions

In pregnancy, a situation where success depends on a large number of variables, one would expect that there would be a large number of causes for pregnancy failure, particularly RSAb. Table 1 outlines the main categories that have been associated

Table 1
Conditions That May Be Associated
with Recurrent Spontaneous Abortion

1.	Anatomical disorders of the female reproductive tract.
2.	Endocrinological abnormalities—ovarian, thyroid, diabetes, and so on.
3.	Reproductive tract infections.
4.	Psychological abnormalities.
5.	Genetic disorders—mother, father, fetus.
6.	Immunological problems: Autoimmunity Materno–fetal immune dysregulation

with RSAb, and there are texts and reviews on these subjects.[11,15] With all these possible causes of RSAb, it is appropriate to ask at the outset what percentage of RSAbs are *not* accounted for by known causes.

Statements have been made that approximately 40% of cases of RSAb have no known etiology.[16] A careful retrospective study of 195 couples with 3 or more failures found that in primary aborters, 66% of the couples had apparent causes for pregnancy failure, whereas 35% of secondary aborters had such identifiable factors.[17] Half of this difference was accounted for by increased anatomical abnormalities in the primary aborting group. Thus, 34% of primary RSAb was idiopathic, whereas 65% of secondary RSAb was associated with unidentified causes. Another study of women with 2 or more losses found that 73% of primary aborters had identifiable risk factors compared with 59% in secondary aborters.[18] Thus, both of these studies agree that about 30–35% of primary aborters have no apparant cause for pregnancy loss. The figure for secondary aborters is 40–60%.

Genetics and RSAb

Before proceeding to immunologic considerations, it is pertinent to review briefly the role of genetic abnormalities in RSAb. In this respect, one should note that the majority of published studies on this subject confine their attention to chromosome

177

structure, although there are obviously many genetic abnormalities that cannot be detected by karyotypic analysis.

In this respect, Gill has long advocated the concept that genetic abnormalities, rather than immunological (or immunogenetic) abnormalities are the major fault in otherwise unexplained RSAb.[19] The experimental basis of his concept comes from animal work with recessive lethal genes. Other collateral evidence cited by Gill are:

1. The increased prevalence of RSAb, congenital anomalies, and cancer in first-, second-, and third-degree relatives of couples with RSAb;
2. The occurrence of RSAb in more than one generation in a family; and
3. The curious but well-known fact that women who abort with one partner may succeed with another.

Gill believes that an apparent association between HLA sharing and RSAb *(see below)* may merely be a marker for some unidentified genetic problem, perhaps a detrimental recessive gene.

Chromosomal Abnormalities

It is widely appreciated that genetic disorders in the parents or in the fetus may lead to fetal wastage. However, there is disagreement as to what kinds of genetic disorders put the pregnancy at risk and what the actual risks may be. This section will review briefly some of the available data that concern identifiable chromosome abnormalities in terms of their influence on RSAb.

Fetal Chromosomal Abnormalities

It is agreed that karyotypic analyses show chromosome abnormalities in about 50% of unselected "random" abortuses, compared with about 0.5% in normal liveborns.[20-23] This figure has been used to suggest that a large proportion of RSAbs might be associated with fetal chromosome anomalies. However, data to support this notion are not easy to find. Ideally, one would want to see karyotypes on all 3 of the abortuses from a primary aborter with 3 losses. Such data are not available, although there is information in RSAb with two miscarriages.

In recurrent spontaneous abortion, one wants genetic data to help in dealing with at least two problems. First, what is the contribution of chromosome abnormalities to RSAb, and second, can karyotypic data help in the management and counseling of couples who have had fetal losses? Intuitively, one might suspect that having one chromosomally abnormal fetal loss would increase the chances of having a subsequent loss of the same kind. This line of thinking assumes that there was a "reason" for the chromosome abnormality in question. That is, the chromosome abnormality was not entirely random; it had a "cause" that might operate in more than one pregnancy in that couple.

Again, data to support this intuitive opinion are difficult to find. Rather surprisingly, the opposite has been reported! Two studies have investigated the risks of subsequent miscarriage, after an index miscarriage was karyotyped. One study showed that the frequency of recurring spontaneous abortion was 16.5% if the previous abortion was karyotypically abnormal, but it was 23% if the previous abortion was karyotypically normal. This improved prognosis in the situation where the prior abortus was karyotypically abnormal was seen if the karyotyped abortion was the first pregnancy or if it had been preceded by deliveries with or without other spontaneous abortions.[20] Another study looked backward and found that the incidence of prior fetal loss was no different in mothers of chromosomally normal abortuses than among mothers of chromosomally abnormal abortuses (25–30%).[23] In still another study of couples with an abortion prior to the karyotyped miscarriage, the frequency of a subsequent abortion (in the third pregnancy) was 40% if the karyotype was normal and 21% if the karyotype was abnormal.[3] A slightly different approach is to ask about the karyotypes of the abortuses when two or more miscarriages are studied. It appears that if the first spontaneous abortion is karyotypically normal, the second tends to be normal, but if the first is abnormal, the second tends to be abnormal.[20,24]

Parental Chromosomal Abnormalities

Most studies are retrospective analyses in which couples have been referred for evaluation after pregnancy losses. Many of these studies include couples with 2 or more spontaneous miscarriages. Some studies also include couples who are secondary aborters and others also include couples where there have been abnormal offspring or untoward perinatal events. In general, these studies do not include "control" couples, so the incidence of abnormalities in RSAb couples is compared to historical controls. The basic question is—what is the likelihood of identifying a chromosome abnormality in either the father or the mother if there have been 2 or more spontaneous abortions? When "major chromosomal abnormalities" are considered, the incidence ranges from 2.9[25] to 10%.[26] ("Major chromosome abnormalities" included reciprocal and Robertsonian translocations, inversions, accessary chromosomes, sex chromosome aneuploidy, and mosaicism.) Other studies reported incidences between these figures.[27,28] If only translocations are considered, the incidence is approximately 2.8%.[29,30] But in women who had only 2 or more miscarriages and no other abnormal perinatal events (e.g., stillbirths or anomalous live births), translocations were found in only 0.3% of the women and 0.4% of the men.[31] Another selective study indicated that in a mixed sample of primary and secondary aborters, there were 6.8% who had chromosome abnormalities, but if one excludes those chromosome abnormalities "of dubious significance" for RSAb (e.g., sex chromosome aneuploidy) only 2.3% of the couples were abnormal.[32] The obvious problem here is that the designation, "of dubious significance," is subject to argument and revision. In addition, one cannot predict fetal chromosome abnormalities by examining parental karyotypes. Of 18 abortuses from 14 couples who were known to carry balanced translocations, only 6 carried unbalanced translocations[33] The other 8 fetuses were either balanced carriers, were karyotypically normal, or had another chromosome anomaly.

In any event, it appears from retrospective studies that demonstrable chromosome abnormalities in habitually aborting couples can be found in 3–10% of such pairs. What is not clear, however, is the incidence of parental abnormalities that are themselves responsible for the miscarriages. Warburton and others believe that retrospective studies tend to overestimate the incidence of chromosome anomalies. Her prospective studies indicate that the importance of parental rearrangements in RSAb is "minute" and the proportion of recurrent abortion with aneuploidy in the parents is "small."[33] A similar opinion is given by Lauritsen.[3]

Immunologic Abnormalities and Recurrent Spontaneous Abortion

Is Immunology Important in Normal Pregnancy?

This question must be considered before one attempts to deal with the relation of immunology to RSAb. It is not an easy question, and many paragraphs in this book have touched on it. Facts pertinent to this question have been gathered from both clinical observation and from animal experimentation. As successful pregnancies occur in highly inbred animal strains, it is clear that these pregnancies can succeed in the absence of traditionally recognized alloreactivity. Nevertheless, there is general agreement that fertility and pregnancy success is *better* when the parents are not genetically identical. Therefore, if there are benefits to outbreeding, they must be viewed as *supplemental,* not essential. (It is also obvious that these supplemental benefits of outbreeding may be genetic as well as immunological.)

Thus, if optimal reproductive performance occurs in the setting of alloreactivity, it may well include some beneficial immunological components, while ensuring that the alloreactive character of the materno–fetal relationship does not lead to fetal "rejection." Thus, the immunogenetic relationship between the mother and the fetus is complex. Perhaps it is a classical example of a "two-handed situation." *On the one hand,* a certain degree of immunogenetic disparity promotes pregnancy success, but *on the other hand,* immunologic reactions may prejudice pregnancy outcome.

The idea that immunological reactivity between mother and fetus is *harmful* comes mainly from studies in autoimmunity. Autoimmune diseases are known to be associated with fetal loss (Chapter 5). Therefore, immunologic reactivity in the mother can cause pregnancy failure. This is highlighted in an unusual but instructive example. In the erythrocyte antigenic system, the rare women with the *p* phenotype make anti-PP P^k antibodies that can cross the placenta. The estimated incidence of early abortion in such cases is 50%.[34–36] Presumably, the maternal antibodies harm the fetus by interacting with the P antigens that are derived from the father.

The idea that immunological reactivity between mother and fetus is *helpful* is a newer idea. This has been called "the immunotrophism hypothesis." It is not certain where it arose but years ago Clarke and Kirby[37] mentioned the possible beneficial effects of maternal anti-paternal antibodies in maintaining genetic polymorphisms in the population as a whole. The immunotrophism hypothesis can be summarized by the statement that the fetus "is immunogenic and evokes a response from the mother that is necessary for successful implantation and growth."[38]

This idea has been entertained recently in a number of places.[39,40] Wegmann gives data to show that in animal systems, placental growth is best in the presence of cytokine growth factors, which in turn are produced or encouraged by T cell activity within the placenta. A failure of such growth-promoting factors would therefore favor pregnancy loss.

In summary, many investigators believe that optimal pregnancy success depends on the presence of beneficial immunotrophic forces and the absence of deleterious immunologic mechanisms exemplified by those seen in autoimmune disease.

Is Immunology Important in RSAb?

This question is also complex. The idea that RSAb may be related to immunology comes from at least four areas. First, as discussed in Chapter 5, overt autoimmune diseases are known to be associated with fetal loss; perhaps there are other more subtle immunologic factors that do not allow a specific diagnosis of autoimmunity that are at fault in RSAb. Second, the beneficial effects of outbreeding may have an immunological basis. Third, there is at least one animal model that seems pertinent to this subject.

The best-studied model of immunologically mediated recurrent pregnancy loss occurs in mice.[6] The basic observation is that CBA females mated with DBA/2 males resorb 30% of the embryos in vivo. A number of interesting facts have been noted. The rate of embryo loss is 10% if the genetic makeups are reversed, i.e., if the females are DBA/2 and the males are CBA. This fact makes one think of immunologically or genetically-mediated pregnancy loss. The two strains differ at the mouse major histocompatibility locus, called H-2; CBA mice are H-2^k and DBA/2 mice are H-2^d. Thus, these strains are genetically different from each other at an important transplantation locus. Furthermore, they also differ by a myriad of non-MHC ("background") genes, whose nature and location are not as well known as the MHC genes. Of most interest to pregnancy immunologists is the fact that the embryo loss rate can be lowered by immunization. However, the benefits of immunization depend on the strain of lymphoid cells used to immunize. Immunization with DBA/2 or CBA cells has no effect, but immunization with BALB/c cells lowers the embryo resorption rate to 5–6%. BALB/c mice also carry the H-2^d MHC genes found in the male partner. However, as immunization with male DBA/2 (H-2^d) cells is not effective, the benefit of immunization with BALB/c cells must be because of gene products *outside* the MHC, i.e., to "background" genes. BALB/c background genes are quite different from both DBA/2 and CBA background genes.

The mechanism of protection by immunization is not clear. Although immunization by various substrains of BALB/c can give varying degrees of protection against embryo less, the development of blocking antibodies and suppressor cells does not correlate with protection.[41] On one hand, it seems extremely useful to have a model of recurrent pregnancy loss in a laboratory animal system where one can carry out detailed experiments looking at a multitude of variables. On the other hand, it is not yet certain that this model has directly and signficantly helped our understanding of RSAb in humans.

Fourth, there are clinical anecdotes that are always intriguing to the practitioner and the investigator, such as the following generic hypothetical scenario. Jane marries John, has 3 pregnancies and delivers 3 children. Jane gets divorced, and marries Bob. Again she has 3 pregnancies but has 3 miscarriages. We then know that Jane can get pregnant and can go to term when John is the father, and she can get pregnant but cannot go to term when Bob is the father. Is there any immunology here? Are there immunological conditions that are "right" for Jane and John but "wrong" for Jane and Bob? If one thinks that advancing maternal age might be a factor, one can reverse the order of the marriages and put the unsuccessful cases first. Although detailed documentation of such scenarios is rare, pregnancy immunologists know that variations on this theme do occur and are extremely thought-provoking.

Histocompatibility Sharing and RSAb

Considerable attention has been paid to the genetic relations between partners in spontaneously aborting couples. It is not certain where the idea arose that habitually aborting couples share more HLA antigens than would be expected on the basis of chance alone. I suspect that the concept got support from several lines of thought. First, it is desirable, from the evolutionary standpoint, to maintain genetic diversity within the population. Therefore, extensive HLA sharing would represent a form of inbreeding and would be undesirable. In this context, RSAb could be considered to be a method of selecting against the reproduction of homozygous individuals. Second, a variation of the above, homozygosity favors the expression of lethal or handicapping recessive genes, and the offspring of HLA-sharing couples might be more likely to carry a lethal gene pair, as some lethal genes have been shown to be MHC-linked.[42,43] Third, there is extensive practical experience that inbred animals do not breed as well as outbred animals. Their litters tend to be smaller and the offspring less robust. Fourth, a possible explanation for why Jane and John have babies whereas Jane and Bob have miscarriages could be less HLA sharing between the first pair and more between the second pair.

A variety of reports have investigated the incidence of HLA sharing between partners in habitually aborting couples and compared this to the incidence of HLA sharing between partners in successful couples. A sample of these studies showed that aborting couples appear to have increased sharing at the HLA-A but not the B locus,[44] at the DR locus,[45] or increased sharing at both A and B loci.[46-48] In papers describing increased HLA-DR sharing, it is disconcerting that a decreased MLR reactivity between aborting as contrasted with successful couples did not correlate with HLA-DR sharing[47,48] as it is the DR locus, which is the major determinant of the strength of the MLR in humans. Another report stressed increased HLA sharing without decreased MLR reactivity in RSAb couples.[49] Other groups have reported no increased HLA sharing.[13,50-54]

In general, the discrepancies between the studies may be accounted for by small sample sizes and inadequately chosen controls. Furthermore, there was usually no distinction made between primary and secondary aborting couples. As mentioned earlier, some investigators believe that primary and secondary RSAb are very different conditions. These investigators believe that increased HLA sharing is more important in primary RSAb, but a recent report indicated increased HLA sharing in both primary and secondary aborters at 3 or more loci with added increased sharing at HLA-A and DQ in primary aborters.[55] Another group, however, did not find increased HLA sharing in either primary or secondary aborting couples.[51]

Another way of looking at this problem is to consider not HLA sharing but *HLA discordance.*[9] After all, the hypothesis that genetic polymorphism is beneficial to the population consider *genetic differences,* which are not exactly the mirror image of genetic similarities. In terms of the hypothesis that it is maternal recognition of paternal antigens that is important, one wants to know what MHC specificities are present in the father that are missing in the mother; presumably these are the source of the fetal immunogenicity (but not if those antigens are present on the noninherited haplotype).

Consider the following couple:

	Woman	*Man*
HLA-A	11, 33	11, 11
HLA-B	8,8	5,8
HLA-DR	1,2	3,4

There is a theoretical maximum of 6 identities or 6 discordances in any pair. In terms of sharing, this man and this woman share HLA-A11, which might be counted as sharing 1 or 2 antigens, since he is homozygous for A-11. They also share HLA B-8, which could be counted as sharing 1 or 2 antigens, because she is homozygous. Thus there might be sharing of 2, 3, or 4 antigens, depending on how the homozygous state is assessed. This is ambiguous. If differences are counted, however, it is quite clear that the man has only 3 specificities that the woman lacks, i.e., B-5, DR3, and DR4. Still, there is an additional source of uncertainty in this example. If one is concerned about homozygosity at any locus, it is not certain whether homozygosity at A or B or DR is significant, or whether it is the woman's or the man's homozygous state that is important.

A still different approach is to analyze closed populations where one would expect to find more HLA sharing than in heterogeneous groups. Extensive studies have been done among the Hutterites, a fairly homogeneous inbred population. An early study in which HLA-A and B were determined indicated that more HLA sharing was associated with a small decrease in fertility; RSAb was not mentioned.[56] A later, more detailed survey emphasized the role of HLA sharing and RSAb. If couples shared HLA DR, there was a 27% incidence of miscarriage, compared with 12% in those not sharing and 9% in those who shared at the A or B loci (all RSAb were secondary).[57] A third survey indicated that HLA sharing was associated with smaller families and longer intervals between the 2nd to 6th births. However, there was no increased incidence of recognized miscarriages.[58] The most recent study of this group by the same investigators indicated that sharing of HLA-B, not HLA-DR, was associated with increased fetal loss.[59] Although inspection of the Hutterite data shows that HLA sharing may be associated with differences in either family size, or intervals between pregnancies or with RSAb, they also show that there were many babies born to couples with HLA sharing, as this community encourages and achieves large families. The possibility that there may be non-HLA genetic influences operating in this inbred population cannot be discounted.

Another approach has been to look at random first pregnancies to determine if the HLA matching or mismatching between parents and children had any effect on the outcome. The distribution of HLA antigens and the degree of HLA sharing was at the expected levels. Two percent of the successful pregnancies had complete HLA-A, -B, and -DR matching between the parents. The conclusion was that successful pregnancies do not show any deviation toward increased fetomaternal incompatibility. However, the incidence of lymphocytotoxic antibodies (LCA's) (postpartum) did correlate with HLA incompatibility, as expected.[60]

Finally, recent intriguing data suggest that a genetic component not directly related to HLA sharing may be important in RSAb.[61] Female sibships in which one woman had RSAb were compared. The incidence of RSAb was higher in siblings where the women shared both parental haplotypes with the index case as compared with sibs who shared only one haplotype.

Consider the following 3 sisters:

	Sib#1	Sib#2	Sib#3
HLA-A	1, 2	1, 2	1, 3
HLA-B	35, 44	35, 44	35, 8
HLA-DR	1, 2	1, 2	1, 3

If sibling #1 is the index case with RSAb, the findings are that RSAb is more common in sibling #2, who is HLA-identical with sibling #1, than in sibling #3, who shares only the haplotype 1-35-1 with the index sibling #1.

The authors concluded that the propensity for RSAb is inherited and that it is associated with the MHC. This idea is intriguing, but it does not indicate whether it is the possession of both haplotypes in siblings #1 and #2 that predisposes to RSAb or whether it is the possession of haplotype 2-44-2 that is at fault—a haplotype that siblings #1 and #2 have but that #3 lacks.

HLA sharing in RSAb is intimately related to the relation of maternal LCAs in normal pregnancy and their possible absence in RSAb. As we have seen, LCAs are made in many (but not all) successful pregnancies. As expected, the more fetomaternal incompatibility, the higher the incidence of LCAs.[60] Conversely, there have been reports that women with RSAb make less LCAs than do successful mothers.[62–64] It is not certain whether this lack of LCAs represents the same phenomenon as a lack of blocking factors (see next section).

Taken together, these and other studies fail to give a clear answer to the question of whether HLA sharing or discordance is important in the etiology of recurrent spontaneous abortion. What is needed is a series of surveys in different populations, with adequate sample size, HLA identification, separation of primary and secondary aborter status, identification of HLA identities and differences, and analysis of the loci of homozygosity.

Suppressor Phenomena in Normal Pregnancy and Recurrent Spontaneous Abortion

A variety of experiments have shown that suppressor influences can be seen locally in the decidua and fetomaternal unit as well as systemically in pregnant women. These include suppression of the MLR and of IL-2 production, in addition to anti-idiotypic responses in the HLA system, all of which have been reviewed earlier in this book. The question now arises as to whether there are any differences in these suppressor mechanisms in recurrent spontaneous abortion, and if so, whether these differences account for the phenomenon of RSAb itself.

An early and provocative report by Rocklin and colleagues described the absence of a blocking factor in RSAb serum.[65] Instead of using the MLR itself as the assay, the investigators measured a product elaborated during the MLR between paternal stimulating PBL and maternal responding PBL. This product was called "migration inhibition factor" (MIF). Its presence was detected by the ability to inhibit the spontaneous migration of third party mononuclear cells in vitro. There were many questions about this assay. The test was difficult to do and has since been abandoned. The precise nature of MIF was not determined, although some investigators favored interferon-γ as the active molecule. The locus and specificity of the blocking was unknown; did it inhibit the paternal cells from stimulating or the maternal cells from responding or from making MIF?[66] Nevertheless, the MIF assay was the principal quantitative in vitro test for delayed type hypersensitivity (DTH) in the precytokine era, and Rocklin and David's group was the pioneer laboratory in this field. Their experiments showed that:

1. MIF was made in MLRs of PBL from either RSAb or successful couples;
2. The serum of multiparous women was able to block MIF production and the blocking factor was IgG;
3. The serum of women with RSAb did not contain material able to block MIF production.

Absorption studies showed that the MIF-blocking ability could be removed by paternal lymphocytes but not by pooled human platelets. Because platelets contain HLA class I antigens, the authors believed that the IgG was not antibody to HLA-A, B, or C but could be antibody to class II MHC (DR). The conceptual scheme elaborated by these experiments was that the

189

normal maternal response to paternal antigens was a DTH response that was potentially harmful to the developing fetus. The successful mother had a circulating IgG that blocked this DTH response. The habitually aborting mother did not have this MIF blocker, and so RSAb was seen as the result of an unopposed or unneutralized maternal antifetal response.

I am not aware that these experiments have been precisely replicated, but the observations raised a great deal of interest. A very similar approach did use the MIF assay but the stimulator material was placental extract rather than paternal PBL.[67] Control PBL did not make MIF in response to stimulation by placental extracts from normal pregnancies. PBL from postpartum "successful" women made MIF to their own placental extract, as did PBL from habitually aborting women. However, plasma from successful women blocked their PBLs MIF production but plasma from aborting women did not. The plasma blocking factor was IgG. Thus, with the difference that placental extract was substituted for husband's PBL, these results are very similar to those of Rocklin et al.[65] Another group indicated that the sera of both primary and secondary aborters failed to block the MLR where the father's cells were stimulators. After 3 blood cell transfusions, however, all cases showed the development of serum blocking factors.[49,68] (The results of the subsequent pregnancies were not reported in this paper.) These results are very provocative because they are in accordance with data that blood transfusions prolong kidney allograft acceptance.[69]

Other approaches have been used. One group claimed that the MLR carried out in pooled serum was depressed in RSAb but the composition of the groups tested was extremely heterogeneous so that clearcut interpretations of the results are difficult.[53] Another study did not find that the MLRs of women with RSAb were any less strong against husband than against pooled stimulators.[49] Singal et al.[70] found that serum from successful pregnancies blocked the MLR between husband stimulator and wife responder cells but this inhibition was not seen with RSAb serum. These results were interpreted to mean that normal pregnancy sera had anti-idiotypic antibodies which blocked the TcR on maternal responding T cells which recognize paternal HLA, (i.e. anti-anti-HLA specificity) and these anti-idiotypes are absent in RSAb.

Cytotoxic, non-cytotoxic and cytotoxic blocking tests have been explored. Although there was a lower incidence of lymphocytotoxic antibodies (LCA) to paternal cells in RSAb compared to successful pregnancies, this may merely reflect a shorter time of exposure to paternal antigens in RSAb [71]. Noncytotoxic antibodies which bound to paternal B cells were found in 11/16 primiparas, 11/11 multiparas, but in only 1/10 RSAb women [63]. Pregnancy serum contained inhibitors of a cytotoxic T cell reaction and this inhibitory property was absent in RSAb serum [72,73]. Again, the distinction between primary and secondary aborters may be important. McIntyre's group found more HLA-A, B, and DR sharing as well as a lack of LCA's and antibody-dependent cellular cytotoxicity (ADCC) in 35 primary aborters and less HLA-A, B, and DR sharing, with 13/15 positive LCA's and 14/15 positive ADCC tests in 15 women with secondary RSAb [8]. However, another laboratory found no correlation between the presence or absence of MLR blocking antibodies and pregnancy outcome [50]. Still a different group found that the ability of serum to block the relevant MLR was higher in multiparas than in women with RSAb (who were similar to nulligravidae). After leukocyte immunization, all 10 women showed increases in serum MLR blocking activity. The investigators believe this was correlated with success in the next pregnancy but the study was small in size and uncontrolled [45]. An evaluation of suppressor cells in the blood of normal pregnancy and RSAb was inconclusive [74].

The concept of TLX polymorphism has been applied to recurrent spontaneous abortion. Indeed, the original TLX exposition [75] suggested that Rocklin's data showing that RSAb sera failed to block MIF production indicated an absence of anti-TA-2 (or anti-idiotype, as the TLX story evolved). Investigators of the TLX system have claimed that anti-TLX antibodies (antibody-1) not neutralized by or complexed with anti-anti-TLX (antibody-2) anti-idiotypes will result in spontaneous abortion.[76] To date, no data to support this concept *specifically in the TLX system* has been put forth.

Finally, there is a dearth of information about the local cellular level that might distinguish successful from RSAb pregnancies. One group did biopsy the uterus in women with incipient sporadic abortion with RSAb and in normal pregnancy. The investigators found more small cells with large granules in normal pregnancy and less of those but more "large granular leukocytes" in spontaneous abortion.[77] Furthermore, cultures of uterine tissue from normal pregnancy produced more suppression of nonspecific mitogen stimulated cultures than did cultures of uterine tissue from aborting pregnancies.

In summary, there are data that indicate that a woman with RSAb does make inhibitory soluble factors able to interfere with maternal-anti-paternal cellular reactions. The nature of these factors is not known, not can this phenomenon be demonstrated in all laboratories. Still, the idea persists that this phenomenon is important in RSAb.

Immunological Therapy for Recurrent Spontaneous Abortion

Rationales for Immunologic Interventions in RSAb

Leukocyte immunotherapy for RSAb appears to have begun about 1980. At least two lines of thought were believed to support this form of treatment. Blood transfusions were known to improve kidney graft survival, although the mechanisms were not clear.[69] Both anti-idiotypic and suppressor T cell activity as well as nonspecific suppression could be important. If kidney graft rejection was similar to fetal loss in RSAb, perhaps cellular infusions would produce a needed blocking material that would promote fetal survival as it did in the case of kidney transplantation. A second rationale was based on the idea that a significant proportion of RSAb couples show increased HLA sharing and that the women fail to make an adequate blocking response to inhibit maternal-anti-paternal incompatibility. As the placenta was purported to have TLX antigens shared by paternal cells, it was believed that immunotherapy to paternal cells would be helpful. The arguments supporting this rationale have been discussed above. The preliminary, uncontrolled results looked very promising.[78,79] I should point out that, even more than the other subjects in this chapter, the question of immunization for RSAb is full of snares and pitfalls for the wary and the unwary alike.

Designing Protocols

The design of any protocols for RSAb immunotherapy will reflect the investigator's assumptions about the etiologies and pathogeneses of RSAb. One must grant that RSAb represents a heterogeneous group of unfortunate women in whom a number of factors may be critical—undetected genetic, infectious, anatomic, endocrinological, or psychological problems may exist, and immunological problems as well. (One assumes that the diagnosable and possibly treatable nonimmunologic aspects will have been taken care of before immunotherapy is started.) How, then, does one proceed? One designs a protocol that will permit the evaluation of immunotherapy for RSAb in a heterogeneous group where neither the frequency of "immunological aborters" nor the efficacy of immunization is known.

At first, it appears simple to envisage what will be needed:
1. The investigator will have, in one treatment center, a sufficient number of women with RSAb of unknown cause who are willing to undergo a randomized, prospective immunotherapy trial;
2. These women will have histories of RSAb that are relatively stereotypical, for instance 3 or more spontaneous abortions; and

3. The women will be sufficiently similar in demographics so that two comparable groups—placebo and treatment—can be gathered.

Even these few considerations turn out to be more complex than they appear at first. Should the trial only contain primary aborters? If, as some groups believe, primary and secondary abortion represent very different immunological phenomena, then either the trial should be limited to primary aborters or, if both primary and secondary aborters are included, they should be separately identified and the numbers in each group should be large enough so that each group can be analyzed statistically to provide some conclusions. Other variables in the RSAb history should be carefully considered. An RSAb history where there is more than one male partner should be grounds for exclusion. Should a positive antiphospholipid antibody test of any kind now become an exclusion criterion? Experience shows that many women with RSAb also have a history of infertility. That is, they not only have trouble *staying* pregnant, but they also have difficulty in *getting* pregnant. Does this "infertility" really represent undetected early pregnancy losses? Should it be weighed in the stratification scheme? What, if anything, should be done to evaluate the male partner from the immunologic standpoint? And, in the newest era of "assisted reproduction," how should one consider women who have had, either with or without success, such procedures as IVF, GIFT, and/or ZIFT? As women with RSAb have an increased incidence of ectopic pregnancies,[80] this factor also needs consideration.

Are there immunological criteria that need to be used in patient selection or stratification? It has been pointed out that LCA are not essential for a successful pregnancy. Sixty-two percent of women with normal pregnancies had no LCA when tested at various times.[71] The fact that 90% of RSAb women had no LCA—a number that looks significantly different from 62%—was accounted for by the fact that many RSAb women aborted before they could develop LCAs. If the woman has lymphocytotoxic antibodies to her husband's cells on preimmunization screening, does this mean that she is already immunized to paternal HLA, and if so, is it to the haplotype on the fetus or to the other, noninherited haplotype? Would further immunization be unnecessary (if not harmful)? Would the same be true if her serum was able to block the MLR where the husband's cells are the stimulator and her cells are the responders?

How large need the study be? In an excellent critical review, Clark and Daya[81] point out that the number needed will, of course, depend on what percentage of RSAb women have immunological problems that can be helped by immunotherapy and how many will have "other" causes for RSAb. (Clark and Daya call these "genetic," but they could be any nonimmunological factors that have assignable success rates in the next pregnancy.) This percentage, of course, is not known—the purpose of the immunotherapy trial is, in part, to determine just what this percentage is. Beforehand, one can only make assumptions as to its size.

Suppose one assumes that 70% of the RSAb women in the trial will be "immunologic," and 30% of the women will have "other" determining factors. Then if one further assumes that 80% of the immunological RSAbs will abort without immunotherapy and that immunotherapy will lower that failure rate to 20%, *and* if one assumes that in the "other" category there will be 70% spontaneous success, *then* one needs 23 treated and 23 placebo patients so that one does not miss the beneficial effects of immunotherapy (but only with a p value of 0.1.).[81] However, if one changes only one variable in that scenario, namely from assuming that 70% of the RSAb in the trial will be immunological to 30%, then one will need 108 patients in each of the placebo and treatment groups in order not to miss a benefit from immunization, but again only with $p \leq 0.1$. Further changes in the assumptions underlying the protocol could raise the number of patients in each group to 240.[81] These are numbers that will probably only be accrued in a cooperative multicenter trial.

In addition, attention must be paid to critical details of the immunization procedure. What cells should be used—husband's or third party donor cells? If one believes that the immunologic problem is "partner-specific," then one would opt for using cells from the husband. If one thinks in terms of other possibly polymorphic systems, e.g., TLX, should one use a third party, and if so, how should that donor be selected? How many cells should be used, and by what route should they be given—intravenous, subcutaneous, or intradermal? How often should injections be given? What constitutes a proper control or placebo injection? Is saline "good enough" or should there be some subtle ingredient that provokes an innocent local reaction and so helps to preserve the "blindness" of the trial? In immunotherapy trials for allergic diseases, some investigators have put a minute amount of histamine into the placebo vials to produce a small and irrelevant wheal-and-flare reaction so that the placebo patients have no reason to believe that they are not getting active material. At least one group giving immunotherapy for RSAb has thought that injections of the woman's own cells is an ideal placebo. If, as seems reasonable (if one ignores the remote possibility of an in vivo correlate of the autologous MLR) (Chapter 1) this injection is indeed a "null" event, it has certain advantages for the *symmetry* of the trial. That is, at each sitting all women and all partners get bled and have cells removed, and all women get an injection of cells, but half of the women are getting autologous cells.

Other questions arise concerning treatment variables. Should cells be injected after a pregnancy is identified? How is one to measure the progress and success of the immunization other than the pregnancy outcome itself? Should one repeatedly test for conversion from the LCA-negative or MLR blocking activity-negative state, and if such conversion occurs, is that a reason to stop immunotherapy?

Immunotherapy trials should be single-variable experiments. That is, the only treatment difference between the two groups should be that one group is receiving foreign cells and the other group is receiving a placebo. How does one insure that no other treatment is in progress? What about the patient whose reproductive endocrinologist is not sure that a luteal phase deficiency has been ruled out and who wants to provide hormonal treatment during the period of immunization?

There are doubtless additional variables and caveats in this area, but the above should suffice to give some idea of the complexity of the situation. Some critics of the immunotherapy approach believe that both the underlying rationale and the results so far are not compelling enough to warrant the continuance of immunotherapy for RSAb.[82]

Results of Immunotherapy for RSAb:
Trials with Nonrandom Controls

Taking all of the above into consideration, one can object beforehand to paying attention to immunotherapy trials that were not prospective, placebo-controlled, and double-blinded with randomly-assigned patients. However, there is considerable experience with less-than-ideal trials, and it is worthwhile summarizing them. Clark and Daya[81] list 7 such attempts. The mean success rate in the next pregnancy was 73.6% (range 40–85%) for the immunized women and 35.4% (range 22–64%) for the historical control groups. The mean of the differences, i.e., the percent of successful next pregnancies in the treated groups minus the percent of successful next pregnancies in the untreated controls was 39.6% (range 2–58%). There are differences in the details of the protocols used in these 7 reports, but the results appear promising. Nevertheless, one should look at the very large variance in the percentages of both successes and failures within the treated groups and within the control groups. In particular, one should note an almost 3-fold range in successful pregnancy rates in the controls, i.e., 22–64%.

Results of Immunotherapy for RSAb:
Trials with Concomitant Random Controls

There are 3 such published trials. In 1985, Mowbray et al. reported the most widely-quoted series.[83] It was a prospective, randomized, double-blinded, placebo-controlled trial, where the placebo was the woman's own PBL. It included primary and secondary aborters and it excluded, among others, Rh⁻ women and those with preexisting antilymphocyte antibodies to the husband's cells. Immunization was given once, the cells being administered by iv, intradermal, and subcutaneous routes. The placebo group had 37% successful pregnancies and the treated group had 77% success. There was no difference between primary and secondary aborters.

Two controlled trials were published in 1991, one from Taiwan[84] and one from Australia.[85] The patients in the first trial were Chinese living in Taiwan and so it was not surprising to find a very significant degree of HLA sharing between aborting partners. If one excludes as too small a group of 11 women who were immunized with third party cells, 49 women received their own cells and 39 received their husband's cells. Of the 49 controls, there was a 62.2% success rate in 37 primary aborters, a 75% success rate in 12 secondary aborters, and an overall success rate of 65.3% Of the 39 immunized women, there was a 76.7% success rate in 30 primary aborters, 88.9% success in 9 secondary aborters, and an overall success rate of 79.5% Although the success rate was higher in the immunized women with both primary and secondary abortion, the differences were not statistically significant. Immunized women did develop an increase in serum blocking factors, but the changes did not correlate with pregnancy outcome. In all, the authors concluded that immunotherapy failed.[84]

The second 1991 trial in Australia included a sequential analysis of 46 couples with 3 or more unexplained miscarriages with the same partner, and no LCAs. Primary and secondary aborters were included, and immunization with husband's cells was done once with a protocol similar to Mowbray's. Sixty-two percent of the immunized women went to term and 76% of those receiving the saline placebo were successful in the next pregnancy. The investigators concluded that immunization was without benefit.[85]

Both of these trials have been criticized.[81] As it is possible to find fault with virtually any clinical trial, it is important to be fair and to try to ascertain if the faults are so severe as to invalidate the trial and its conclusions. The criticisms of these trials do not appear to this reviewer to be devastating enough to cause us to ignore the negative results. To be sure, larger groups of patients would be desirable, and might have permitted the uncovering of a beneficial effect of immunotherapy that could not be seen in the trials as they now stand.

Even so, the negative results, like the results of the uncontrolled trials, do deserve scrutiny, and the outstanding factor that requires attention is the success rate in the placebo-treated patients. In the uncontrolled trials, this percentage ranged from 22 to 64%; in controlled studies, it was 65% in the Taiwan trial, 76% in the Australian report, but only 37% in the London experience. This is such a wide range that one is puzzled. Is the difference a result of different basic biological phenomena in disparate ethnic groups, or of different criteria for patient inclusion or exclusion, of better obstetrical diagnosis or treatment, or even of psychological variables or "placebo effects"? Clark and Daya review the results of one randomized controlled and one unrandomized study that appear to show that psychotherapy is successful in treating RSAb. It should be noted that the untreated control groups had very low success rates (26 and 36%) compared with 84 and 85% success in the groups receiving psychotherapy. These low control success rates are very similar to those seen in the London trial where immunotherapy appeared to be successful, but very different from the very high success rates seen in the controls in the Taiwan or Australian trials, where immunotherapy appeared to have failed.

Experience at the University of Colorado

It is appropriate, I believe, to outline briefly our experience in immunization for TSAb over the past 6 years. We have treated approximately 98 women in whose cases there has been sufficient elapsed time to judge the outcome.

Selection of Patients

Women have been referred from practitioners in private practice and from the University of Colorado. Most have been primary aborters with three or more spontaneous miscarriages with the current partner. A few have been primary aborters close to or beyond the age of 35 with only two abortions. A few have been secondary aborters. All women are screened for lymphocytotoxic antibodies against the husband's PBL. If the test is positive (as happens rarely), they are not immunized. Couples are HLA typed at the HLA-A, B, and Dr loci. Women with positive anticardiolipin tests are excluded.

Immunization

Immunization is carried out twice at monthly intervals. Buffy coat cells from 25 mL blood are concentrated and injected intradermally into 10–30 sites on the upper arm. (The blood has been screened in the blood bank as if it were to be transfused in the usual fashion.)

Post-Immunization Testing

Post-immunization testing consists of determining whether the woman developed leukocytotoxic antibodies against her husband's cells or if her serum produced 40% inhibition of a series of mixed leukocyte cultures where her cells, her husband's cells, and random third-party cells were used as stimulators and/or responders. If either the LCA or the MLC blocking is positive, no further immunization is given. If both tests are negative, a third immunization is given. If this fails, a few women are reimmunized with third-party cells.

Results

About 60% of the women converted serologically. There is not a close correlation between the development of LCA or MLR blocking factors and a successful pregnancy. The "success rate" depends on how one calculates the pregnancy outcomes. Forty-three women had successful pregnancies, 30 women had spontaneous abortions, and there were 2 fetal deaths. This provides a success rate of 56%. Four of the women who had spontaneous abortions went on to a successful pregnancy; this gives a success rate of 47 out of 79 pregnancies (60%). In addition, there were 2 ectopic pregnancies, and 23 women failed to become clinically pregnant. Four women had two successful pregnancies but each woman is counted only once. Among the successful pregnancies were 3 premature infants who were otherwise normal. Except for one baby with mild congenital heart disease there were no birth defects.

Comments

This was a study of 98 women without controls. During the course of immunizations, a very large number of questions arose, which make me wonder how a truly satisfactory controlled immunization trial could be conducted. It is instructive to consider some of these problems, even though thorough statistical analyses of our data have not been carried out. Each problem constitutes a potential variable thath might or might not be important.

HETEROGENEITY OF PREGNANCY HISTORIES. Each habitually aborting couple has a unique history. There are primary and secondary aborters, and there may be more than one partner for the primary or secondary aborters. Most women have had 3 or more RSAbs, but some women near or beyond the age of 35 have been immunized after two miscarriages. It is difficult to say to a 36-year-old woman with "only" two miscarriages; "Come back after you have had a third spontaneous abortion and we will let you enter the program." Difficulty becoming pregnant is almost as common as difficulty staying pregnant. Excess HLA sharing is not often seen, but on occasion, couples may share 3 of 6 HLA-A,

HLA-A, B, and DR antigens. Conversely, there are couples in which the husband has 3 or fewer antigens that the wife does not have. Low-level positive ANA tests are not rare, even in the absence of overt autoimmune disease or anticardiolipin antibodies.

CONCOMITANT TREATMENT VARIABLES. Many women, during or following their immunization, receive hormonal supplementation for conditions such as luteal phase deficiency. It is unreasonable and unrealistic to try to eliminate this variable from the treatment process. In addition, couples are now seeking various forms of assisted reproduction in those cases where there is fertility delay. These maneuvers include in vitro fertilization, artificial insemination, and GIFT and ZIFT procedures. It may seem inappropriate at first sight to use immunotherapy—a strategy devised to *maintain* pregnancy—for couples having difficulty achieving pregnancy. If, however, one considers that many cases of apparent fertility delay may really represent very early pregnancy losses, then the rationale becomes clearer for using immunotherapy in situations that include IVF and GIFT.

Other students of RSAb may well add may more variables, hazards, and confounding aspects to the above discussion. Thus, physicians who are thinking of developing controlled immunization trials for RSAb need to keep a multitude of considerations in mind. They represent a daunting set of hurdles, indeed.

*Other Immunological Approaches
to the Treatment of RSAb*

The trials discussed above have used treatment with leukocytes, a treatment based on the idea that the mother's response to antigens on the surface of fetal cells should be modulated. Other approaches have also been tried. Pooled human gamma globulin given intravenously (IVIG) is undergoing trials.[86] This modality has been proven to be effective in the treatment of autoimmune thrombocytopenia and Kawasaki disease and is suspected of being beneficial in other immunologic conditions not related to frank immunoglobulin deficiency.[87] The mechanism underlying the benefit in these diseases is not certain, but the presence of anti-idiotypic antibodies in the general population raises the possibility that IVIG provides anti-idiotypic immunoglobulin that might be lacking in some people. If RSAb is associated with a failure to make anti-idiotypes in the MHC system, then IVIG may represent a sensible approach to treatment. A few cases of RSAb with antiphospholipid antibodies have been treated successfully with IVIG.[88] The rationale for such treatment includes the possibility that IVIG might contain anti-immunoglobuins capable of inhibiting the harmful effects of the APL antibodies. Seminal plasma vaginal suppositories are being tried, as a means of immunizing against TLX antigens, which are putatively present in seminal fluid.

Hazards of Immunotherapy for RSAb

No treatment is medicine is without hazard, so risk-benefit considerations are important. IVIG material is carefully screened for its content of infectious agents and appears to be quite safe. The preparation process excludes or inactivates hepatitis B and HIV viruses. Newer batches will undoubtedly be screened for hepatitis C.[89] Although IVIG is mostly of the IgG isotype, it does contain some IgA and therefore could cause production of anti-IgA in those 1/500-1/750 people who are IgA deficient. If these anti-IgA antibodies are of the IgE isotype, anaphylaxis may ensue.[89]

The possible hazards of paternal or third party leukocyte immunization require more thought. Hill[82] has presented a long list of dangers, ranging from graft-vs-host disease in mother or baby, transmission of infectious diseases, malformation in the fetus, sensitization to platelets or erythrocytes, and enhanced abortion, infertility, or autoimmunity. It suffices at this point to say that no instances of the above have been clearly proven to have occurred secondary to the immunization procedure and to have been injurious, although such untoward events are always possible. Leukocyte donors are screened for infectious disease as are any blood transfusion donors. One would expect that an

RSAb woman would already have considerable conjugal exposure to infectious agents present in the husband, but this, of course, would not apply in the case of third party immunization. One hazard that was not mentioned is the very sensitization to the husband's HLA antigens, which is the objective of leukocyte immunotherapy. If immunization is successful in raising HLA sensitization, then the women would thereby become very poor risks for organ transplantation (e.g., receiving a kidney from the husband). Even after considering the statistical unlikelihood of this event, HLA sharing is still only arguably present in RSAb couples and is rarely of such a magnitude to make the husband a "good match" for kidney donation to the wife even without immunization. There have been unsystematic and anecdotal reports of intrauterine growth retardation after immunization for RSAb. However, it is not at all clear that control populations were free of this hazard, and so the issue has not been resolved.[15]

Summary

This chapter has concerned the possible role(s) of immunology in the etiology, pathogenesis, and therapy of RSAb. There is a great deal of conflicting opinion on all aspects of this topic.

1. The immunological processes that may help maintain normal pregnancy are not well known. In particular, it is not certain whether a successful pregnancy requires local or systemic immunological responses, perhaps of a suppressor or blocking nature.
2. The definitions and determinations of incidence and prognosis in RSAb are not clear enough. These questions need to be addressed again in the light of newer means of assessing early pregnancy loss. The differences between primary and secondary abortion need to be clarified.
3. Possible immunological irregularities that may be responsible for RSAb have not been ascertained with sufficient accuracy. This includes possible increased sharing of

HLA (or other putatively polymorphic antigenic entities), and the presence or absence of maternal suppressor or blocking influences. The bulk of the recent data do not support the concept that excessive HLA sharing between habitually aborting partners is important in RSAb.

4. Immunotherapeutic approaches to RSAb require attention. Even if one grants the existence of immunological roles in RSAb, therapy trials need to be planned and executed on a larger scale than heretofore, with a standardization of the protocol design and clarification of the ways of assessing the relevant immunological variables. The current information is discordant and does not allow one to decide whether immunotherapy for RSAb is effective or not.

References

1. Stirrat GM: Recurrent Miscarriage. I. Definition and epidemiology. *Lancet* 1990; 336: 673–675.
2. McIntyre JA, Coulam CB, Faulk WP: Recurrent spontaneous abortion. *Am J Reprod Immunol* 1989; 21: 100–104.
3. Lauritsen JG: Genetic aspects of spontaneous abortion. *Dan Med Bull* 1977; 24: 169–188.
4. Little AB: There's many a slip 'twixt implantation and the crib. *N Engl J Med* 1988; 319: 241–242.
5. Wilcox AJ, Weinbert GR, O'Connor JF, et al.: Incidence of early loss of pregnancy. *N Engl J Med* 1988; 319: 189–194.
6. Clark DA, Chaout G: What do we know about spontaneous abortion mechanisms? *Am J Reprod Immunol Microbiol* 1989; 19: 28–38.
7. Coulam CB, Moore SB, O'Fallon WM: Association between major histocompatibility antigen and reproductive performance. *Am J Reprod Immunol Microbiol* 1987; 14: 54–58.
8. McIntyre JA, McConnachie PR, Taylor CG, et al.: Clinical, immunologic, and genetic definitions of primary and secondary recurrent spontaneous abortions. *Fertil Steril* 1984; 42: 849–855.

9. Coulam CB, McIntyre JA, Faulk WP: Reproductive performance in women with repeated pregnancy losses and multiple partners. *Am J Reprod Immunol* 1986; 12: 10–12.

10. Reginald PW, Beard RW, Chapple J, et al.: Outcome of pregnancies progressing beyond 28 weeks in gestation in women with a history of recurrent miscarriage. *Br J Obstet Gynecol* 1987; 94: 643–648.

11. Stirrat GM: Recurrent miscarriage. II. Clinical associations, causes, and management. *Lancet* 1990; 336: 728–733.

12. Roman E: Fetal loss rates and their relation to pregnancy order. *J Epidemiol Community Health* 1984; 38: 29–35.

13. Houwert-de Jong MH, Termijtelen A, Eskes TKAB, et al.: The natural course of habitual abortion. *Eur J Ob Gyn Reprod Biol* 1989; 33: 221–228.

14. Knudsen UB, Hansen V, Juul S, et al.: Prognosis of a new pregnancy following previous spontaneous abortions. *Eur J Ob Gyn Reprod Biol* 1991; 39: 31–36.

15. Beard RW, Sharp F: Early pregnancy loss: Mechanisms and treatment. *Royal Coll Obstet Gynaecol* 1988; 351–354.

16. Beer AE: New horizons in the diagnosis, evaluation and therapy of recurrent spontaneous abortion. *Clin Obstet Gynecol* 1986; 13: 115–124.

17. Stray-Pedersen B, Stray-Pedersen S: Etiologic factors and subsequent reproductive performance in 195 couples with a prior history of habitual abortion. *Am J Obstet Gynecol* 1984; 148: 140–146.

18. Harger JH, Archer DF, Marchesp SG, et al.: Etiology of recurrent pregnancy losses and outcome of subsequent pregnancies. *Obstet Gynecol* 1983; 62: 574–581.

19. Gill III TJ: Influence of MHC and MHC-linked genes on reproduction. *Am J Hum Genet* 1992; 50: 1–5.

20. Boue J, Boue A, Lazar P: Retrospective and prospective epidemiological studies of 1500 karyotyped spontaneous human abortions. *Teratology* 1975; 12: 11–26.

21. Simpson JL, Bombard A: Chromosomal abnormalities in spontaneous abortion: Frequency and genetic counseling, in Bennett MJ, Edmonds DK (eds): *Spontaneous and Recurrent Abortion*. Oxford, Blackwell Scientific; 1987: 51–76.

22. Kline J, Stein Z: Epidemiology of chromosomal anomalies in spontaneous abortion: Prevalence, manifestation and determinants, in Bennett MJ, Edmonds DK (eds): *Spontaneous and Recurrent Abortion.* Oxford, Blackwell Scientific; 1987: 29–50.

23. Hassold T, Chen N, Funkhouser J, et al.: A cytogenetic study of 1,000 spontaneous abortions. *Ann Hum Genet* 1980; 44: 151–178.

24. Kajii T, Ferrier A: Cytogenetics of aborters and abortuses. *Am J Obstet Gynecol* 1978; 131: 33–38.

25. Tharapel AT, Tharapel SA, Bannerman RM: Recurrent pregnancy losses and parental chromosome abnormalities: A review. *Br J Obstet Gynaecol* 1985; 92: 899–912.

26. Sachs ES, Jahoda MGJ, van Hemel JO, et al.: Chromosome studies of 500 couples with two or more abortions. *Obstet Gynecol* 1985; 65: 375–378.

27. Fryns JP, Kleczkowska A, Kubien E, et al.: Cytogenetic survey in couples with recurrent fetal wastage. *Hum Genet* 1984; 65: 336–354.

28. Campana M, Serra A, Neri G: Role of chromosome aberrations in recurrent abortion: A study of 269 balanced translocations. *Am J Med Genet* 1986; 24: 341–356.

29. Gadow EC, Lippold S, Otano L, et al.: Chromosome rearrangements among couples with pregnancy losses and other adverse reproductive outcomes. *Am J Med Genet* 1991; 41: 279–281.

30. Kleinhout J, Madan K: Repeated abortions and chromosome analysis, in Hafez ESE (ed): *Spontaneous Abortion.* Boston, MTP Press; 1984: 143–152.

31. Simpson JL, Meyers CM, Martin AO, et al.: Translocations are infrequent among couples having repeated spontaneous abortions but not other abnormal pregnancies. *Fertil Steril* 1989; 51: 811–819.

32. Castle D, Bernstein R: Cytogenetic analysis of 688 couples experiencing multiple spontaneous abortions. *Am J Med Genet* 1988; 29: 549–556.

33. Warburton D, Strobino B: Recurrent spontaneous abortion, in Bennett MJ, Edmonds DK (eds): *Spontaneous and Recurrent Abortion.* Oxford, Blackwell Scientific; 1987: 193–213.

34. Cantin G, Lyonnais J: Anti-PP1Pk and early abortions. *Transfusion* 1983; 23: 350–351.

35. Shirey RS, Ness PM, Kickler TS, et al.: The association of anti-P and early abortion. *Transfusion* 1987; 27: 189–191.

36. Race RR, Sanger R: *Blood Groups in Man*, Oxford, Blackwell Scientific Publishing Co.; 1975: 139.

37. Clarke B, Kirby D: Maintenance of histocompatibility polymorphisms. *Nature* 1966; 211: 999–1000.

38. Scott JR, Rote NS, Branch DW: Immunologic aspects of recurrent abortion and fetal death. *Obstet Gynecol* 1987; 70: 645–656.

39. Klopper A: Pregnancy proteins and hormones in the immune response of pregnancy, in Stern CMM (ed): *Immunology of Pregnancy and its Disorders*. Dordrecht, Kluwer Academic Publishers; 1989: 91–113.

40. Wegmann TG: Placental immunotrophism: The idea and evidence, in Chaouat G (ed): *The Immunology of the Fetus*. Boca Raton, CRC Press, Inc.; 1990: 180–185.

41. Bobe P, Chaouat G, Stanislawski M, et al.: Immunogenetic studies of spontaneous abortion in mice. II. Antiabortive effects are independent of systemic regulatory mechanisms. *Cell Immunol* 1986; 98: 477–485.

42. Gill III TJ: Immunogenetics of spontaneous abortions in humans. *Transplantation* 1983; 35: 1–6.

43. Awdeh ZL, Raum D, Yunis EJ, et al.: Extended HLA/complement allelic haplotypes: Evidence for a T/t-like complex in man. *Proc Natl Acad Sci USA* 1983; 80: 259–263.

44. Gerencer M, Kastelan A, Drazancic A, et al.: The HLA antigens in women with recurrent abornal pregnancies of unknown etiology. *Tissue Antigens* 1978; 12: 223–227.

45. Takakuwa K, Kanazawa K, Takeuchi S: Production of blocking antibodies by vaccination with husband's lymphocytes in unexplained recurrent aborters: The role in successful pregnancy. *Am J Reprod Immunol Microbiol* 1986; 10: 1–9.

46. Beer AE, Quebbeman JF, Ayers JWT, et al.: Major histocompatibility complex antigens, maternal and paternal immune responses and chronic habitual abortions in humans. *Am J Obstet Gynecol* 1981; 141: 987–999.

47. McIntyre JA, Faulk WP: Recurrent spontaneous abortion in human pregnancy: Results of immunogenetical, cellular, and humoral studies. *Am J Reprod Immunol* 1983; 4: 165–170.
48. Thomas ML, Harger JH, Wagener DK, et al.: HLA sharing and spontaneous abortion in humans. *Am J Obstet Gynecol* 1985; 151: 1053–1057.
49. Unander AM, Lindholm A, Olding LB: Blood transfusions generate/increase previously absent/weak blocking antibody in women with habitual abortion . *Fertil Steril* 1985; 44: 766–771.
50. Sargent IL, Wilkins T, Redman CWG: Maternal immune responses to the fetus in early pregnancy and recurrent miscarriage. *Lancet* 1988; 2: 1099–1104.
51. Cauchi MN, Tait B, Wilshire MI, et al.: Histocompatibility antigens and habitual abortion. *Am J Reprod Immunol Microbiol* 1988; 18: 28–31.
52. Caudle MR, Rote NS, Scott JR, et al.: Histocompatibility in couples with recurrent spontaneous abortion and normal fertility. *Fertil Steril* 1983; 39: 793–798.
53. Lauritsen JG, Kristensen T, Grunnet N: Depressed mixed lymphocyte culture reactivity in mothers with recurrent spontaneous abortion. *Am J Obstet Gynecol* 1976; 125: 35–39.
54. Oksenberg JR, Pesitz E, Amar A, et al.: Mixed lymphocyte reactivity non-responsiveness in couples with multiple spontaneous abortions. *Fertil Steril* 1983; 39: 525–529.
55. Ho H-N, Gill III TJ, Hsieh R-P, et al.: Sharing of human leukocyte antigens (HLA) in primary and secondary recurrent spontaneous abortions. *Am J Obstet Gynecol* 1990; 163: 178–188.
56. Ober CL, Martin AO, Simpson JL, et al.: Shared HLA antigens and reproductive performance among Hutterites. *Am J Hum Genet* 1983; 35: 994–1004.
57. Ober CL, Hauck WW, Kostyu DD, et al.: Adverse effects of human leukocyte DR sharing on fertility: A cohort study in a human isolate. *Fertil Steril* 1985; 44: 227–232.
58. Ober C, Elias S, O'Brien E, et al.: HLA sharing and fertility in Hutterite couples: Evidence for prenatal selection against compatible fetuses. *Am J Reprod Immunol Microbiol* 1988; 18: 111–115.

59. Ober C, Elias S, Kostyu DD, et al.: Decreased fecundability in Hutterite couples sharing HLA-DR. *Am J Hum Genet* 1992; 50: 6–14.

60. Jazwinska EC, Kilpatrick DC, Smart GE, et al.: Fetomaternal HLA compatibility does not have a major influence on human pregnancy except for lymphocytotoxin production. *Clin Exp Immunol* 1987; 69: 116–122.

61. Christiansen OB, Riisom K, Lauritsen G, et al.: Association of maternal HLA haplotypes with recurrent spontaneous abortions. *Tissue Antigens* 1989; 34: 190–199.

62. Unander AM, Olding LB: Habitual abortion: Parental sharing of HLA antigens, absence of maternal blocking antibody, and suppression of maternal lymphocytes. *Am J Reprod Immunol* 1983; 4: 171–178.

63. Power DA, Catto GRD, Mason RJ, et al.: Evidence for protective antibodies to HLA-linked paternal antigens. *Lancet* 1983; ii: 701–704.

64. Johnson PM, Barnes RMR, Harti CA, et al.: Determinants of immunological responsiveness in recurrent spontaneous abortion. *Transplantation* 1984; 38: 280–284.

65. Rocklin RE, Kitzmiller JL, Carpenter CB, et al.: Maternal-fetal relation: Absence of an immunologic blocking factor from the serum of women with chronic abortions. *N Engl J Med* 1976; 295: 1209–1213.

66. Rocklin RE, Kitzmiller JL, Kaye MD: Immunobiology of the maternal-fetal relationship. *Ann Rev Med* 1979; 30: 375–404.

67. Stimson WH, Strachan AF, Shepherd A: Studies on the maternal immune response to placental antigens: Absence of a blocking factor from the blood of abortion-prone women. *Br J Obstet Gynecol* 1979; 86: 41–45.

68. Unander AM, Cindholm A: Transfusions of leukocyte rich erythrocyte concentrates: A successful treatment in selected cases of habitual abortion. *Am J Obstet Gynecol* 1984; 154: 516–520.

69. van Rood JJ: Pretransplant blood transfusion: Sure! But how and why? *Transplant Proc* 1983; 15: 915–916.

70. Singal DP, Butler L, Liao S-K, et al.: The fetus as an allograft: Evidence for antiidiotypic antibodies induced by pregnancy. *Am J Reprod Immunol* 1984; 6: 145–151.

71. Regan L, Braude PR: Is paternal cytotoxic antibody a valid marker in the management of recurrent abortion? *Lancet* 1987; ii: 1280.

72. Fizet D, Bousquet J, Piquet Y, et al.: Identification of a factor blocking a cellular cytotoxicity reaction in pregnant serum. *Clin Exp Immunol* 1983; 52: 648–654.

73. Fizet D, Bousquet J: Absence of a factor blocking a cellular cytotoxicity reaction in the serum of women with recurrent abortions. *Br J Obstet Gynaecol* 1983; 90: 453–456.

74. Fiddes TM, O'Reilly DB, Centrulo C, et al.: Phenotypic and functional evaluation of suppressor cells in normal pregnancy and in chronic aborters. *Cell Immunol* 1986; 97: 407–418.

75. Faulk WP, Temple A, Lovins RE, et al.: Antigens of human trophoblasts: A working hypothesis for their role in normal and abnormal pregnancies. *Proc Natl Acad Sci USA* 1978; 75: 1947–1951.

76. McIntyre JA: In search of trophoblast-lymphocyte crossreactive (TLX) antigens. *Am J Reprod Immunol Microbiol* 1988; 17: 100–110.

77. Michel M, Underwood J, Clark DA, et al.: Histologic and immunologic study of uterine biopsy tissue of women in incipient abortion. *Am J Obstet Gynecol* 1989; 161: 409–414.

78. Taylor C, Faulk WP: Prevention of recurrent abortion with leukocyte transfusion. *Lancet* 1981; ii: 68–70.

79. Taylor C, Faulk WP, McIntyre JA: Prevention of recurrent spontaneous abortions by leukocyte transfusion. *J Royal Soc Med* 1985; 78: 623–627.

80. Fedele L, Acaia B, Parazzini F, et al.: Ectopic pregnancy and recurrent spontaneous abortion: Two associated reproductive failures. *Obstet Gynecol* 1989; 73: 206–208.

81. Clark DA, Daya S: Trials and tribulation in the treatment of recurrent spontaneous abortion. *Am J Reprod Immunol* 1991; 25: 18–24.

82. Hill JA: Immunological mechanisms of pregnancy maintenance and failure: a critique of theories and therapy. *Am J Reprod Immunol* 1990; 22: 33–42.

83. Mowbray JF, Gibbings C, Liddell H, et al.: Controlled trial of treatment of recurrent spontaneous abortion by immunisation with paternal cells. *Lancet* 1985; 4/27/85 issue: 941–943.

84. Ho H-N, Gill TJ, Hsieh H-J, et al.: Immunotherapy for recurrent spontaneous abortions in a Chinese population. *Am J Reprod Immunol* 1991; 25: 10–15.

85. Cauchi MN, Lim D, Young DE, et al.: Treatment of recurrent aborters by immunization with paternal cells—controlled trial. *Am J Reprod Immunol* 1991; 25: 16–17.

86. Coulam C, Peters A, McIntyre J, et al.: The use of IVIG for the greatment of recurrent spontaneous abortion, in Imbach P (ed): *Immunotherapy with Intravenous Immunoglobulins*. London, Academic Press; 1991: 395–400.

87. Dwyer JM: Manipulating the immune system with immune globulin. *N Engl J Med* 1992; 326: 107–116.

88. Wapner RJ, Cowchuck FS, Shapiro SS: Successful treatment in two women with antiphospholipid antibodies and refractory pregnancy losses with intravenous immunoglobulin. *Am J Obstet Gynecol* 1989; 161: 1271–1272.

89. Buckley RH, Schiff RI: The use of intravenous immune globulin in immunodeficiency diseases. *N Engl J Med* 1991; 325: 110–117.

Epilogue

The Answers?

The original stimulus for this book was my long-standing fascination with the immunological paradox of pregnancy—*What mechanisms have developed that allow a genetically and immunologically foreign fetus to survive to term?* The proximate impetus for getting the facts on paper was my involvement in a controversial topic, i.e., immunotherapy for spontaneous recurrent abortion.

The resolution of the paradox is much clearer than it was just 10 years ago. However, I am not convinced that the problem has been completely solved, because of the complexities of the immune system, and of materno–fetal interactions.

The most striking advance has been the discovery of the nonpolymorphic HLA-G system on the trophoblast at the feto–maternal interface. The development of such an apparently inert MHC molecule would seem to be a clever move on the part of evolutionary processes to negate the possibility of maternal alloreactivity against paternal antigens on the fetus. Thus, although Peter Medawar's number one explanation of the paradox was *anatomic* separation of the fetus from the mother, HLA-G appears to represent an *immunologic* separation.

However, HLA-G, serving as an inert barrier may not be the entire solution to the paradox. As mentioned earlier in this book, biological control pathways are generally complex, often involving redundant and overlapping systems as "fail-safe" mechanisms. It is easy to see that the control (or prevention) of maternal immunological reactions potentially harmful to the fetus is such an important evolutionary concept that more than one mechanism may have developed. Thus, some questions come to mind.

If an inert, immunologically "null" interface is needed, why have *any* MHC molecule at all on the syncytiotrophoblast? The system might, perhaps just as easily, have evolved to a syncytiotrophoblast with *no MHC* present. Unless, of course, HLA-G has some positive or beneficial function at the interface. That possibility remains to be explored.

What is the significance of a complement component, i.e., membrane cofactor protein (MCP) on the trophoblast? It too, like HLA-G, appears nonpolymorphic. But, also like HLA-G, it is a part of the immunological system. Is the complement system important in materno–fetal interactions and, if so, how does it function?

What is the significance of materno–fetal alloreactivity, for example, the presence of lymphocytotoxic antibodies, when it is present? Is it an epiphenomenon, of no survival value to mother or fetus? If not, is it helpful or harmful? How carefully is it regulated, for instance by anti-idiotypic responses at the T or B cell level? And if such regulation is a common occurrence, what are the biological benefits (and perhaps costs) to the pregnant woman?

What seems quite certain is that the answers to these and other questions will provide further fascinating insights into the immunologic paradox of human pregnancy.

Index